Baillière's
CLINICAL
HAEMATOLOGY

INTERNATIONAL PRACTICE AND RESEARCH

Baillière's

CLINICAL

HAEMATOLOGY

INTERNATIONAL PRACTICE AND RESEARCH

Volume 2/Number 1
January 1989

Aplastic Anaemia

E. C. GORDON-SMITH MA, FRCPath, FRCP
Guest Editor

Baillière Tindall
London Philadelphia Sydney Tokyo Toronto

Baillière Tindall 24–28 Oval Road,
W.B. Saunders London NW1 7DX

The Curtis Centre, Independence Square West,
Philadelphia, PA 19106–3399, USA

1 Goldthorne Avenue
Toronto, Ontario M8Z 5T9, Canada

Harcourt Brace Jovanovich Group (Australia) Pty Ltd,
32–52 Smidmore Street, Marrickville, NSW 2204, Australia

Exclusive Agent in Japan:
Maruzen Co. Ltd. (Journals Division)
3–10 Nihonbashi 2-chome, Chuo-ku, Tokyo 103, Japan

ISSN 0950-3536

ISBN 0-7020-1281–5 (single copy)

Baillière's Clinical Haematology is published four times each year by Baillière Tindall.
Annual subscription prices are:

TERRITORY	ANNUAL SUBSCRIPTION	SINGLE ISSUE
1. UK	£40.00 post free	£18.50 post free
2. Europe	£50.00 post free	£18.50 post free
3. All other countries	Consult your local Harcourt Brace Jovanovich office for dollar price	

The editor of this publication is Katherine Hinton, Baillière Tindall,
24–28 Oval Road, London NW1 7DX.

Baillière's Clinical Haematology was published from 1972 to 1986 as
Clinics in Haematology.

Typeset by Phoenix Photosetting, Chatham.
Printed and bound in Great Britain by Mackays of Chatham PLC, Chatham, Kent.

Contributors to this issue

ANDREA BACIGALUPO MD, Head of Transplant Unit, Department of Haematology, San Martino Hospital, Viale Benedetto XV, 10, 16132 Genova, Italy

RICHARD CHAMPLIN MD, Associate Professor of Medicine, Director, Transplantation Biology Program, Division of Hematology/Oncology, UCLA Center for Health Sciences, Los Angeles, CA 90024, USA.

DAVID I. K. EVANS MA, MB, BChir, FRCPEd, DCH, Consultant Haematologist, Royal Manchester Children's Hospital, Pendlebury, Manchester M27 1HA, UK; Lecturer (part-time) in Child Health; University of Manchester, Manchester, UK.

ELIANE GLUCKMAN Professor, UFGM, Hôpital Saint Louis, 1 Avenue Claude Velle-faux, 75475 Paris Cedex 10, France.

EDWARD C. GORDON-SMITH MA, FRCPath, FRCP, Department of Haematology, St. George's Hospital Medical School, Cranmer Terrace, Tooting, London SW17 0RE, UK.

ALISON LOUISE JONES MB, ChB, MRCP, Clinical Research Fellow, Royal Marsden Hospital, Sutton, Surrey, UK.

GARY KURTZMAN MD, Division of Haematology, Department of Internal Medicine, Stamford University School of Medicine, Stamford, CA 94025, USA.

LUCIO LUZZATTO MD, FRCP, FRCPath, Professor of Haematology, Royal Post-graduate Medical School, University of London; Consultant Haematologist, Hammersmith Hospital, Du Cane Road, London W12, UK.

JOHN LEIGH MILLAR BSc, MSc, PhD, MRCPath, Team Leader, Section of Medicine, Institute of Cancer Research, Royal Marsden Hospital, Clifton Avenue, Belmont, Surrey, UK.

CATHERINE NISSEN-DRUEY MD, Associate Professor, Medical Faculty, University of Basel, University Hospital, Petersgraben 4–8, 4031 Basel, Switzerland.

BRUNO ROTOLI MD, Associate Professor of Haematology, University of Napoli, Second Medical School, Via S. Pansini 5, 80131 Napoli, Italy.

TIM R. RUTHERFORD MA, PhD, Department of Haematology, St. George's Hospital Medical School, Cranmer Terrace, Tooting, London SW17 0RE, UK.

NEAL YOUNG MD, Chief, Cell Biology Section, Clinical Hematology Branch, National Heart, Lung and Blood Institute, Bethesda, Maryland 20892, USA.

Table of contents

RECENT ISSUES

September 1987
Blood Rheology and Hyperviscosity Syndromes
G. D. O. LOWE

December 1987
Chronic Myeloid Leukaemia
J. M. GOLDMAN

FORTHCOMING ISSUES

April 1989
Iron Chelating Factors
C. HERSHKO

July 1989
Platelet Disorders
J. CAEN

Foreword

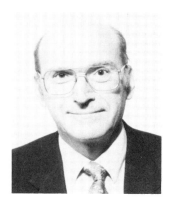

The non-malignant disorders of haemopoiesis which may be linked by the concept of haemopoietic precursor cell failure have proved to be a fascinating meeting point between clinical pathology and experimental physiology, between disease and the theories of normal haemopoiesis. In this volume we have tried to emphasize the relationship between what happens in the patient and the observations made in the laboratory on normal bone marrow development, which may help in the understanding of both normal and abnormal situations. It has to be said that production of this volume has coincided with a period of enormous change and excitement in the study of haemopoiesis and its control; a change which is still continuing with the introduction of growth factors and inhibitors in the laboratory and the early attempts at using them in the clinical setting. Likewise, the possible role of viruses in these non-malignant disorders and the genetic basis of the inherited diseases are being studied with the techniques of molecular biology which multiply almost monthly.

The book is not only an exposition of the known scientific basis of bone marrow failure, but is also an attempt to describe the natural history of these somewhat uncommon disorders and to discuss the effectiveness of currently available treatment.

The hope is always that a better understanding of scientific principles will lead to better treatment or perhaps prevention of disease. This hope is not always fulfilled, at least in the short term, but without the understanding, improved therapy will rarely be achieved.

The invited authors in this book have all made distinguished contributions in the scientific and clinical study of bone marrow failure and have stuck to the task of seeking explanations for the clinical observations. I am grateful to them.

E. C. GORDON-SMITH

1

Aplastic anaemia—aetiology and clinical features

E. C. GORDON-SMITH

It is just 100 years since Paul Ehrlich described the first case of acquired aplastic anaemia in what he thought was a variant of pernicious anaemia (Figure 1). Over the next 75 years recognition of the disease as a separate entity from pernicious anaemia and from malignant disease slowly evolved. The association with exposure to drugs was recognized and the idiosyncratic nature of the disorder appreciated, in that the vast majority of patients exposed to these drugs did not develop aplastic anaemia. There was still considerable confusion about the diagnosis which was often based on peripheral blood findings only in the absence of adequate bone marrow material. In the older literature many cases of pancytopenia are described as aplasia, many of which would now be recognized as myelodysplasia or associated with malignant disease. Refinement in diagnostic techniques has occurred over the past 25 years or so, first with the introduction of adequate trephine biopsies and subsequently with the development of in vitro culture techniques. Cytogenetic analysis has also played its part.

The interest in aplastic anaemia, rare though it is, was spurred on by the introduction of improved methods of support and treatment; first, the introduction of allogeneic bone marrow transplantation (Storb et al, 1974) and subsequently the evident benefit of treatment with antilymphocyte globulin (Speck et al, 1977; Champlin et al, 1983). Despite this upsurge of interest its pathogenesis remains enigmatic (Camitta et al, 1982; Thomas and Storb, 1984). Even whether the diagnosis may be applied to a relatively homogeneous group or whether it represents only the end-stage of a number of different processes is in doubt. Aplastic anaemia remains a frustrating and intriguing disorder and all too often a devastating one.

DEFINITION

The functional definition of aplastic anaemia is the failure of haemopoietic stem cells to proliferate and differentiate in the absence of any predictable cause. However, since it is impossible to recognize or measure stem cell function in humans, such a definition remains speculative and cannot indicate whether the failure of stem cell function is the result of an intrinsic defect or the consequence of changes in the microenvironment of the stem cells.

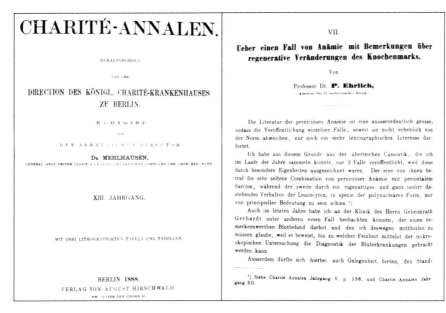

Figure 1. Frontispiece and first page of Paul Ehrlich's description of aplastic anaemia (courtesy of Professor R. Ihle).

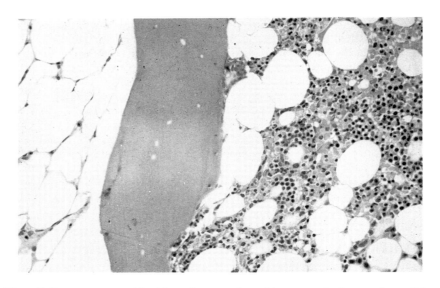

Figure 2. Bone marrow trephine biopsy from a patient with severe aplastic anaemia: acellular marrow space on the left of the bone trabeculum and cellular area on the right with prominent erythroid islands.

Definition of aplastic anaemia therefore rests on the haematological and clinical findings, mainly of a negative nature. Whilst the diagnosis is straightforward in the majority of cases, there are a growing number of variants which can only be classified as aplastic anaemia from the evolution of the disease.

The peripheral blood shows pancytopenia involving the red cell, granulocytic and platelet series. There is anaemia with a relative reticulocytopenia, reduction in all granulocytic cells and thrombocytopenia. The lymphocyte count is more variably reduced and the total lymphocytes may be normal, more commonly in children than in adults.

The bone marrow shows replacement of normal haemopoietic tissue by fat cells though islands of haemopoietic tissue may remain (Lewis, 1965; Kansu and Erslev, 1976) so that both bone marrow aspirate and trephine are essential for the diagnosis and more than one sample may have to be obtained (Figure 2). The reticulin content of the bone marrow is reduced commensurately with the degree of hypocellularity. Malignant cells are absent from the bone marrow.

Clinical features should show no abnormal physical findings apart from those associated with the results of pancytopenia. There should be no history of exposure to agents which predictably cause marrow suppression and the family history should not indicate the possibility of genetic factors. It is conventional to separate cases with paroxysmal nocturnal haemoglobinuria (PNH) from idiosyncratic acquired aplastic anaemia, though the two disorders overlap (Lewis and Dacie, 1967); the acidified serum lysis test (Ham's test) should be negative.

HAEMATOLOGY

There are no specific features of the haematological findings but certain aspects increase the probability of the diagnosis and assist in the differential diagnosis. In the peripheral blood the red cells may show macrocytosis, particularly if there is some residual haemopoietic function. There is often anisocytosis, sometimes quite marked, but the presence of teardrop poikilocytes should raise the possibility of PNH or a myeloproliferative disorder. Neutrophil morphology is normal apart from an increase in the size and number of granules, producing the so-called 'toxic granulation' appearance. The neutrophil alkaline phosphatase score is raised, falling if PNH clones develop. The eosinophils and basophils are reduced together with the neutrophils, and granulocyte precursors are not seen. The morphology of the remaining peripheral blood cells is normal although there may be an increase in activated lymphocyte forms. Immunophenotyping of the remaining lymphocytes usually demonstrates a normal distribution (Elfenbein et al, 1979) except for the finding of a slight proportional increase in activated suppressor cells indicated by a rise in the $CD8^+$ positive, Tac^+ positive cells (Zoumbos et al, 1985; see Chapter 3). In the majority of patients the reduction in numbers in the three cell series is similar in proportion, indicating a general failure of differentiation. In some cases there may be relative sparing of one cell line or particular reduction in another. Most commonly it is the platelets and the red cells which are reduced, most prominently in the initial stages, though it is the reduction in neutrophil numbers which determines the prognosis (see below). The greatest difficulty in diagnosis arises when only one cell series is reduced and it may be necessary to follow the course of the disease over a period of months or even years before arriving at a definite conclusion.

In the bone marrow the changes which lead to the diagnosis are also mainly dependent on negative findings. The bone marrow aspirate may demonstrate the typical fatty fragments and hypocellular trails of typical aplastic anaemia. Occasionally a cellular remnant of marrow may be aspirated, in which case the fragments appear cellular or even hypercellular and normal haemopoietic cells appear in the cell trails. Even in these cases the number of megakaryocytes is reduced. Macrophage activity appears prominent in many cases of aplastic anaemia, particularly in the early stages of the disease. Erythrophagocytosis and even haemophagocytosis may be seen and macrophages contain fat and haemosiderin granules. The remaining haemopoietic cells have a normal appearance or show only mild dysplastic changes. Non-haemopoietic cells, including lymphocytes, plasma cells and mast cells together with the macrophages, may be prominent but it is not possible to determine if there is a true increase in these remaining cells. Malignant cells or an increase in blast cells are not seen.

The bone marrow trephine biopsy confirms the overall hypocellularity of the marrow with the replacement of haemopoietic tissue by the fat cells. A number of different patterns of remaining cells may be seen, of which the significance is not clear. Islands of apparently normal haemopoietic tissue may remain, as shown in Figure 2. Although these islands of cells appear superficially normal there is often a relative decrease in megakaryocyte content. Within these islands of cells groups of erythroid or granulocytic precursors forming distinct entities suggest attempts at regeneration but cultures of granulocytic precursors, colony-forming unit–granulocyte macrophage (CFU-GM) indicate a considerable reduction in progenitor cells. Lewis (1965) showed that these remaining patches of haemopoietic tissue did not influence the outcome of the disease, which depends most obviously on peripheral blood count.

The meaning of the patterns of remaining non-haemopoietic cells has also stimulated discussion. The remaining cells consist of fibroblasts, lymphocytes, plasma cells and macrophages. A painstaking study by Te Velde and Haak (1977) suggested that there were three main patterns in these remaining cells. In the first pattern such cells were sparse and the marrow was generally completely hypocellular. In the second there was a diffuse appearance to these 'chronic inflammatory' cells and in the third, islands of lymphoid or inflammatory tissue remained. In that study it appeared that the diffuse pattern of chronic inflammatory cells had a worse prognosis than those with islands of lymphoid tissue but responded better to antilymphocyte globulin. These findings were not confirmed in a later study (Sale et al, 1987) and the significance of the non-haemopoietic cells remains obscure. No significant changes in the populations of lymphocytes remaining in the aplastic marrow compared to normal have yet been demonstrated.

Short-term culture of bone marrow cells from patients with aplastic anaemia demonstrates a reduction in all types of committed precursor cells (Haak et al, 1977; Bacigalupo et al, 1980; Sullivan et al, 1980). The morphology of those colonies which do grow appears to be normal and an increase in cluster formation is not seen. Culture of stromal cells has produced conflicting results. Fibroblast colonies appear to be functionally normal (Gordon and Gordon-Smith, 1983) but there may be a decrease in the total number. Fibroblast colonies from patients with aplastic anaemia may produce fat cells spontaneously in the absence of additional hydrocortisone (Gordon and Gordon-Smith, 1981). This may reflect the concentration of various growth factors in the blood, most of which seem to be increased in aplastic anaemia (Nissen et al, 1983). Serum from patients with aplastic anaemia usually increases colony formation from normal bone marrow, suggesting an excess of growth factors. Direct measurement of erythropoietin shows this to be markedly increased in aplasia, as is granulocyte macrophage colony-stimulating factor (GM-CSF).

Ferrokinetic studies using ^{59}Fe or ^{52}Fe reflect the involvement of the erythropoietic system. Iron clearance is prolonged, though not usually to the extent seen in pure red cell aplasia. Iron utilization is decreased most markedly in the most severely affected patients. ^{52}Fe scanning may show patches of remaining erythropoietic marrow but generally the uptake of iron is poor within the marrow system, with most of the iron accumulating in the liver. Ferrokinetic studies may be helpful in identifying cases of aplastic anaemia where the marrow aspirate and trephine have produced relatively cellular samples.

AETIOLOGY OF APLASTIC ANAEMIA

An association between the development of aplastic anaemia and previous exposure to drugs or industrial chemicals has been recognized for many years (Jick, 1977) but since there is no test to demonstrate that a particular drug was responsible for an individual case of aplastic anaemia, such an association is based upon epidemiological evidence associated with the temporal relationship between exposure and the development of aplasia. Viruses, particularly non-A non-B hepatitis viruses, are also thought to be responsible for a proportion of cases of aplastic anaemia. In about 70% of patients with aplastic anaemia no obvious aetiological agent can be suspected.

DRUGS AND APLASTIC ANAEMIA

A wide variety of drugs have been implicated in aplastic anaemia (Niewig, 1973; Heimpel and Heit, 1980) but in the majority of instances the number of cases for individual drugs is small and epidemiological evidence weak (International Agranulocytosis and Aplastic Anemia Study, 1986). Chloramphenicol is perhaps the best documented and most notorious of the drugs which may cause aplastic anaemia. Chloramphenicol was introduced into clinical practice in 1949 and it was suggested at that time on the basis of its chemical similarity to amidopyrine that it might cause blood dyscrasias (Smadel and Jackson, 1947). Amidopyrine was known to cause agranulocytosis and on occasions aplastic anaemia. In 1950, the first case of chloramphenicol-induced aplastic anaemia was described in a patient who received a prolonged course of chloramphenicol for osteomyelitis (Rich et al, 1950). Further reports followed over the next few years and it became apparent that chloramphenicol was more likely to produce aplastic anaemia than agranulocytosis.

In the majority of these early cases chloramphenicol was used for good clinical reasons and in standard antibacterial doses. Cases were reported in which the dose of chloramphenicol given was low and was discontinued some time before the aplasia developed. Later still, cases of aplastic anaemia were reported following the use of chloramphenicol eyedrops (Abrams et al, 1980; Fraunfelder et al, 1982; Fraunfelder and Bagby, 1983); this has led to the notion that aplastic anaemia following exposure to chloramphenicol is not dose-dependent. It is however difficult on epidemiological grounds to confirm this statement. A number of cases of aplastic anaemia following exposure to chloramphenicol eyedrops seems to be about 15 in the total world literature. In some of these instances the association is weak if based on temporal grounds. The incidence of aplastic anaemia in patients exposed to chloramphenicol eyedrops or ointment cannot be much greater than the background incidence. On the other hand prolonged or repeated courses of chloramphenicol do seem to provoke a higher incidence (Williams et al, 1973), of the order of 1/25 000 of patients exposed.

How chloramphenicol produces aplastic anaemia is unknown. The antibacterial action of chloramphenicol depends upon its action in binding to the large subunit of bacterial ribosomal RNA (Hahn and Gund, 1975; Werner et al, 1975) and inhibiting protein synthesis. Chloramphenicol does not bind to the equivalent subunit in eukaryotic ribosomal RNA coded for by nuclear DNA. Protein synthesis is inhibited in bacteria by chloramphenicol but not in eukaryotic cells.

Chloramphenicol will bind to ribosomal RNA coded for by mitochondrial DNA in mammalian cells (Wheeldon and Lehninger, 1966). Chloramphenicol does produce a dose-dependent inhibition of haemopoiesis, particularly affecting the erythroid series (Hara et al, 1978; Yunis et al, 1980) and leading in some instances to the development of ringed sideroblasts. This inhibition of haemopoiesis is reversible and predictable and does not seem to be the basis for prolonged acquired aplastic anaemia. Mehta and colleagues (1987) investigated the possibility that patients who developed aplastic anaemia following exposure to chloramphenicol had a mutation or polymorphism in the mitochondrial DNA which might make them more susceptible to the action of chloramphenicol than the majority of the population. In one case of recovered aplastic anaemia they were able to demonstrate a polymorphism in the mitochondrial DNA coding for ribosomal RNA which was in a similar region to known polymorphisms in other species which confer resistance to the action of chloramphenicol (Kearsey and Craig, 1981). However this polymorphism was not found in other patients with chloramphenicol-induced aplastic anaemia and has occasionally been found in the normal population.

The role of such genetic factors remains obscure. Genetic factors in the susceptibility to chloramphenicol have been suggested by the finding of more than one member of a family who developed aplastic anaemia following exposure to the drug (Nagro and Maver, 1969) but the nature of the blood disorder was not typical of classical acquired aplastic anaemia.

Thiamphenicol, an analogue of chloramphenicol, has a similar antibacterial action but a lower incidence of aplastic anaemia. Cases have however been reported following thiamphenicol (De Renzo et al, 1981) and the drug has had a much smaller usage, so the incidence of blood dyscrasia is unknown.

Phenylbutazone and its analogue, oxyphenbutazone, have also been widely implicated in the production of blood dyscrasias including aplastic anaemia (Heimpel et al, 1976; Inman, 1977). These pyrazolones share some structural similarities to chloramphenicol and to amidopyrine. The incidence of aplastic anaemia following exposure to phenylbutazone is probably similar to that seen with chloramphenicol (Lancet, 1986).

Other non-steroidal anti-inflammatory drugs have also been reported as causing aplastic anaemia. Benoxaprofen (Opren) was associated with a number of cases before its withdrawal from the market on the basis of toxicity. Indomethacin (Canada and Burka, 1968; Lancet, 1986) and sulindac have also been recorded as being associated with aplastic anaemia but the risk factor for these drugs seems to be less than for phenylbutazone or chloramphenicol (International Agranulocytosis and Aplastic Anemia Study, 1986). Although cases of aplastic anaemia have been reported in association with other non-steroidal anti-inflammatory drugs including aspirin (Wijna et al, 1966), their aetiological role must still remain in doubt.

Gold-induced aplastic anaemia is well documented (Kay, 1973; Baldwin et al, 1977). How gold salts induce aplastic anaemia is unknown. Neutropenia or thrombocytopenia are not uncommon following the use of gold salts in rheumatoid arthritis and persistence with the treatment in the face of neutropenia is more likely to lead to aplastic anaemia. In those patients who have recovered from gold salt-induced aplastic anaemia it is possible to demonstrate the presence of gold within the bone marrow up to several years after recovery.

Investigation of the aetiology and pathogenesis of aplastic anaemia is further complicated by the observation that there may be a delay of 1–6 months between exposure to the supposed aetiological agent and the development of pancytopenia. In a few instances, it is possible to document normal or nearly normal blood counts following cessation of treatment and before the pancytopenia develops (Gordon-Smith, 1979). Exposure to a putative agent more than 6 months before development of the aplasia reduces the index of suspicion.

CHEMICAL EXPOSURE AND APLASTIC ANAEMIA

A prolonged idiosyncratic aplastic anaemia has been reported in association with a number of industrial practices, including the aniline dye industry and those industries where organic solvents are widely used. The effects of benzene on bone marrow activity has been most extensively studied (Gardner, 1987) and in the majority of cases exposure to benzene produces a dysplastic syndrome rather than true aplastic anaemia (Aksoyer et al, 1972).

Chromosome damage may also be observed. In many industries benzene was withdrawn as a solvent and replaced by non-aromatic solvents such as Stoddard's solvent. Even so, cases of aplastic anaemia have been described in workers using these solvents.

VIRUSES AND APLASTIC ANAEMIA

The role of viruses in the pathogenesis of aplastic anaemia is considered in detail in Chapter 4. Non-A non-B hepatitis appears to be the best established associated disorder, though Epstein-Barr virus infection (Sanka et al, 1987) and influenza A have also been reported as preceding aplastic anaemia. Most patients who develop aplastic anaemia following hepatitis have severe peripheral blood pancytopenia and therefore a poor prognosis, but when the outcome is compared with idiopathic aplastic anaemia of similar severity there is no difference in outcome.

INCIDENCE OF APLASTIC ANAEMIA

The incidence of aplastic anaemia in developed temperate countries is probably of the order of 3–6 per million of population per annum (Wallerstein et al, 1969; Szklo et al, 1985). Estimates which put the incidence rather higher than this (Bottiger and Bottiger, 1981) probably included a number of myelodysplastic cases, particularly in the older age group. In the Far East, China and Japan the incidence appears to be rather higher than in the West (Aoki et al, 1980), perhaps because of the higher prevalence of hepatitis, the more widespread use of chloramphenicol and the extensive use of insecticides (Young et al, 1986). The difference does not appear to be genetic since people from these populations who move to the West have the same rate of attack by the disease as the indigenous population.

In most series there seems to be a preponderance of males, perhaps because of the increased risk of industrial exposure to potential toxins.

There appear to be two peaks in age distribution of acquired aplastic anaemia. The incidence of the disease decreases between the ages of about 20 and 40 and then rises again in old age (Szklo et al, 1985). In the latter group there may be some confusion with the myelodysplastic syndromes. This age distribution may well reflect attack by viruses and exposure to unidentified toxic agents. In children it is of course important to identify those patients who have a congenital aplastic anaemia.

CLASSIFICATION OF APLASTIC ANAEMIA

The concept of severe disease

Patients with aplastic anaemia die as a consequence of the failure of the bone marrow. Without blood products support the majority of patients would die within a short period of time (Lynch et al, 1975). The introduction of blood transfusion and in particular, of platelet transfusion, has considerably modified the natural history of the disease. Before the introduction of allogeneic bone marrow transplantation by E. Donnall Thomas and colleagues in Seattle, the only treatment for the disease was the support of blood products and availability of antibiotics for treatment of infection. The introduction of androgens by Shahidi and Diamond in 1959 also modified the outlook, though only for a short while (Li et al, 1969). About 50% of patients treated with androgens and blood products support died within 3–6 months of the diagnosis (Williams et al, 1973), immaterial of whether the aplasia was drug-induced, postviral or idiopathic. The major prognostic criteria lay in the peripheral blood count (Lewis, 1965) which led to the notion that patients with aplastic anaemia could be divided into two groups, those with severe aplastic anaemia (SAA) who had a 10% chance of recovery and those with non-severe aplastic anaemia where recovery approached 50%. Using a multisystem analysis, Camitta and colleagues (1975) defined SAA, as shown in Table 1. These criteria have had an

Table 1. Criteria for severe aplastic anaemia (from Camitta et al, 1982).

Peripheral blood
Pancytopenia with at least two of the following:
    Neutrophils $<0.5 \times 10^9/l$
    Platelets $<20 \times 10^9/l$
    Reticulocytes $<1\%$ (corrected for haematocrit)

Bone marrow
Assessed on trephine biopsy
    Severely hypocellular: $<25\%$ normal
or
    Moderately hypocellular: 25–50% normal with less than 30% remaining cells haemopoietic

important influence on analysis of response to different therapies as it has become customary to compare the effects of different treatments, for example immunosuppression and bone marrow transplantation, in patients with similarly severe disease.

Subsequent improvement in support measures, particularly the availability of human leukocyte antigen (HLA)-matched platelet transfusions and new antibiotic treatment, has improved the outlook for patients who do not receive bone marrow transplantation. Analysis of collected European data of patients treated with immunosuppression or bone marrow transplantation by the European Bone Marrow Group has shown that there is a group of patients with SAA who are particularly at risk unless they receive an

HLA-matched bone marrow transplant. These are patients with SAA in whom the neutrophil count is particularly reduced, below 0.2×10^9/l, and who have evidence of infection at the time of treatment. These patients are considered to have very severe aplastic anaemia (VSAA). The results of this analysis are given in more detail in Chapter 2.

MANAGEMENT OF APLASTIC ANAEMIA

Support measures

The major support measures for patients with aplastic anaemia are the provision of blood products, protection from external and internal sources of infection and treatment of infection when it does arise. The way in which blood products are used may affect subsequent treatment if the patient goes on to receive a bone marrow transplant. At the initial presentation these effects should be borne in mind, even though the patient may present requiring urgent blood transfusion. Two important factors which influence the outcome of bone marrow transplantation are sensitization of the patient to platelet transfusion (Storb and Deeg, 1986) and the development of cytomegalovirus (CMV) infection in the post-transplant period (Meyers et al, 1986). Initial procedures which should be carried out at presentation are the determination of the severity of the disease, the availability or otherwise of an HLA-matched sibling donor and the CMV status of the patient. Patients with severe aplastic anaemia treated by bone marrow transplantation who are CMV-negative should receive CMV-negative blood products throughout the period when they require transfusions irrespective of the CMV status of the donor (Grob et al, 1987). Therefore, all patients who may be going on to such treatment should initially be transfused with CMV-negative blood products, where possible, until the CMV status of the patient has been determined. Clearly the measurement of CMV antibodies as well as hepatitis B and hepatitis A status is urgent for such patients. If the patient is CMV-negative, he or she should where possible continue to receive CMV-negative blood products even if the potential donor is CMV-positive, since there is evidence to suggest that CMV pneumonitis is less likely in CMV-negative recipients receiving a transplant from a CMV-positive donor than in CMV-positive recipients (Grob et al, 1987).

Sensitization to blood products leading to anti-HLA antibodies or specific platelet antibodies may be avoided or reduced by giving granulocyte-depleted transfusions (Eernisse and Brand, 1981) and HLA-matched platelets. At present it is not feasible to manage the majority of patients with such ideal blood products but the introduction of in-line filters to remove the majority of white cells from red cell or platelet transfusion may improve the situation in the future (Kickler et al, 1988). For the present, patients who present with thrombocytopenia or anaemia requiring urgent correction should receive the appropriate CMV-negative transfusions, only avoiding transfusions from family members which may lead to specific sensitization, thus greatly increasing the risk of graft rejection.

Once the initial assessment of the patient's disease and prospects for therapy are completed it may become apparent that he or she will require long-term blood product support. The level of haemoglobin maintained in any individual patient will depend to a considerable extent upon his or her symptomatology and activity. The majority of patients may be maintained with haemoglobin levels between 7 and 9 g/dl but others, perhaps with more active lifestyles, require a higher level. Problems of iron overload rarely occur in these patients and the problems of neutropenia and thrombo-cytopenia make the early use of subcutaneous desferrioxamine undesirable.

Platelet transfusions are required by most patients, particularly those with severe aplastic anaemia. Cerebral haemorrhage is a major cause of death in patients with aplastic anaemia and it may be advisable to use regular prophylactic platelet transfusions rather than using platelets to correct haemorrhagic symptoms, though this is debatable (Kelton and Ali, 1973; Slichter, 1980; Klingemann et al, 1987). During the initial management of the patient it usually becomes apparent whether the failure of platelet production is going to require regular platelet transfusions or not. Apart from the advantages of preventing severe haemorrhage, prophylactic platelet transfusions have the added advantage of logistical planning, particularly if HLA-matched platelets are required. Whether HLA-matched platelets can be used from the beginning of support will depend upon their availability from the blood transfusion service. In most cases, HLA-matched platelets probably cannot be provided for all patients who are at risk from sensitization. Random donor platelets therefore have to be used until the patient becomes sensitized (Klingemann et al, 1987). Sensitization is indicated by a failure of platelet increment after transfusion of random donor platelet and regular measurements of anti-HLA antibodies should be made so that HLA-compatible platelets may be used if such antibodies develop (Herzig et al, 1975). Sensitization by platelets is not inevitable; it occurs in about 50% of patients (Dutcher et al, 1981a), but small numbers of transfusions may produce sensitization in susceptible patients (Dutcher et al, 1981b).

Increased platelet transfusion support is required during treatment with antilymphocyte globulin and throughout the bone marrow transplant procedure.

The use of granulocyte transfusion is debatable but in general it has little place in the management of aplastic anaemia. Prophylactic granulocyte transfusions are not cost-effective (Rosenshein et al, 1980), even if the logistical problems can be overcome. There may be some purpose in using granulocyte transfusions to help eradicate a superficial localized infection or a proven Gram-negative sepsis which does not respond to appropriate antibiotics (Strauss, 1983) but transfusion of granulocytes, particularly in the presence of amphotericin or pulmonary complications, may lead to an exacerbation of the consolidation.

Prevention of infection

Patients with aplastic anaemia are at risk from infection which proliferates in the presence of neutropenia. Unlike patients with leukaemia treated with chemotherapy, the remainder of the immune system in the aplastic anaemia patient is intact. The rate of infection is lower in aplastic patients (Keidan et al, 1986) than in patients with acute leukaemia (Bodey et al, 1982) but the chronicity of the disease makes death from infection more likely. Measures must be devised to protect the patient from serious bacterial or fungal infection over a prolonged period of time but which are compatible with management and may include outpatient care.

Patients who have a neutrophil count greater than $0.5 \times 10^9/l$ have a low risk of bacterial or fungal infection. Patients with a neutrophil count between 0.2 and $0.5 \times 10^9/l$ have an increased risk of infection which is mainly apparent during therapy with antilymphocyte globulin or corticosteroids. Patients with a neutrophil count of less than $0.2 \times 10^9/l$ have a greatly increased risk of infection and require special long-term consideration.

Protective measures are designed to avoid acquired bacterial or fungal infection, mainly during periods of hospitalization. The major source of bacterial infections in patients with aplastic anaemia is from potentially pathogenic organisms in the gastrointestinal tract, the respiratory passages (Schimpff et al, 1972; Meyers, 1986) and from invasive procedures such as the insertion of a central venous catheter. Patients with a neutrophil count of less than $0.5 \times 10^9/l$ should be managed throughout hospital care in protective isolation. Minimal standards of care should include an isolation room, preferably with filtered air to avoid infection by fungi—particularly *Aspergillus*—and separate toilet and washing facilities. Most hospital infections are transmitted from the hands or clothing of staff caring for the patients so all such staff should wash with an antiseptic handwash effective against fungi as well as bacteria and should remove clothing likely to be infected from other patients and wear a clean gown.

Infection from enteric organisms can be reduced by giving the patient non-absorbable antibiotics effective against aerobic organisms within the gut (Van Saene and Stoutenbeek, 1987). Antifungal agents are also required. Various regimens have been devised, of which a combination of framycetin, colistin and nystatin is one which seems to be well tolerated without producing unacceptable diarrhoea. Oral hygiene with chlorhexidine mouthwash and amphotericin lozenges is also important. Oesophageal candidiasis is not uncommon and a nystatin suspension should regularly be taken four times daily.

The question of food for patients with chronic neutropenia is also difficult to answer. Ideally patients should receive food of low bacterial content, that is to say food which is freshly cooked. Patients are advised to avoid salads and fruit which may be a potential source of pathogens but it is not possible to determine the risk of pathogenic organisms causing problems from such sources. The risk is probably higher in hospitals than in the home environment.

Treatment of fever

In the severely neutropenic patient the time interval between the development of the first signs of infection in the fever and the onset of shock and renal failure may be too short to allow the usual procedures for identifying responsible organisms. Such severe and rapid infections are mostly the result of Gram-negative infection, particularly by *Pseudomonas* species or *Klebsiella*, though *Candida* septicaemia can produce a similar picture. Gram-positive infections, commonly with *Staphylococcus epidermidis*, are less rapidly progressive and most of the antibiotic regimens given when patients with severe neutropenia develop infections are designed to combat Gram-negative septicaemia.

When fever develops in these patients appropriate samples for the identification of the causative organism should be taken and once this has been accomplished the patient commenced on intravenous antibiotics. The antibiotic schedule chosen will depend on a knowledge of the distribution of local pathogens. These local pathogens may have been identified from an initial baterial screening of the patient or from a knowledge of antibiotic-resistant hospital organisms. Gentamicin and piperacillin is a suitable initial combination if gentamicin-resistant organisms are known to be absent from the environment. Other combinations of aminoglycoside and ureido-penicillin may be devised for particular circumstances. Ceftazidime used as a single agent is also effective (Gaya, 1986). If these fevers fail to respond to these measures after 24 h Gram-positive cover should be introduced in the form of vancomycin. Vancomycin should also be used prophylactically to cover the period of insertion of a central venous catheter. The antibiotic regimen should of course be modified in the light of subsequent identification of a particular pathogen.

The identification of fungal infections in severely neutropenic patients may be difficult and the introduction of antifungal agents, particularly amphotericin, is always a difficult decision. Infection with *Candida* should be considered probable if *Candida* has been isolated from two or more sites during surveillance screening. Fungal infection of the sinuses may also occur in these patients. In general fungal infections are more likely in the neutropenic patient who has been treated for a prolonged period of time with broad-spectrum antibiotics or received corticosteroids, but fungal infections may occur early in the disease and it is a mistake not to consider the possibility simply because the clinical history is short. Patients with severe neutropenia whose fever persists after 3 or 4 days of broad-spectrum antibiotics covering both Gram-negative and Gram-positive organisms should receive a trial of amphotericin. In the presence of a proven fungal infection or where there is a high index of suspicion amphotericin should be started at the highest possible dose rather than escalating slowly, as is usually recommended. Following the test dose amphotericin should be introduced at 0.5 mg/kg body weight/day, increasing as rapidly as possible to 1 mg/kg/day. This latter dose may have to be reduced slightly because of nephrotoxicity.

TREATMENT OF APLASTIC ANAEMIA

The treatment of aplastic anaemia is discussed in detail in Chapter 5. The first important decision is whether bone marrow transplantation or immuno-suppression is the appropriate first form of therapy. If immunosuppression is the better or only form of treatment the patient, relatives and staff must be warned that recovery is slow and that hospital-oriented care may be required for a year or more. Since it may be said that patients with aplastic anaemia die as a result of failure of supportive care, constant vigilance is required as well as anticipation of problems to avoid this outcome as far as possible.

Selection for bone marrow transplantation

Patients under the age of 20 with SAA as judged by the criteria given in Table 1 who have an HLA-matched sibling donor should be considered for allogeneic bone marrow transplantation as the first therapeutic option. Patients under 50 who have VSAA should also be considered as candidates for bone marrow transplantation if a suitable donor is available. Other patients should receive a trial of antilymphocyte globulin even if an HLA-matched sibling donor is available. For those with a matched sibling donor transplantation should be considered if there is no response to antilympho-cyte globulin after 3 months.

Patients without an HLA-matched sibling donor who fail to respond to one or more courses of antilymphocyte globulin present a major problem. Isolated reports of the beneficial effects of cyclosporin suggest that it may be appropriate to try this drug (Stryckmans et al, 1984). Current trials in Europe involving cyclosporin with or without antilymphocyte globulin may eventually demonstrate how effective this form of treatment will be (Frickhofen et al, 1986). The use of matched unrelated donors for bone marrow transplantation in aplastic anaemia has so far proved disappointing and must be considered highly experimental (Hows et al, 1986).

COURSE OF APLASTIC ANAEMIA

It will be apparent that the course of aplastic anaemia is greatly modified by support procedures and by the effects of treatment. Nevertheless, a certain pattern may be discerned. In the majority of patients the presenting blood count and bone marrow finding give a good indication of the severity of the disease and the likely problems which will be encountered before recovery occurs. In other patients who present with non-severe aplastic anaemia or in whom there is preservation of one cell line, observations over the initial 2 or 3 weeks will indicate whether the findings are stable or whether the disease is going to progress into the SAA group. Such careful consideration is impor-tant since it may modify the treatment option considered.

Response to immunosuppressive treatment is slow and the first indication of this response may be an increase in the mean cell volume of the red blood cells. There may be a stabilization of blood counts at a level below normal, the patient no longer requires transfusion support and his or her neutrophils have improved so that spontaneous infection becomes less likely. This unstable state may go on to complete remission, may relapse with the return of aplastic anaemia or may show evidence of clonal disorders such as PNH, myelodysplastic state or even rarely progress to acute leukaemia. This instability of the recovered marrow means that the patient who recovers from aplastic anaemia should be followed for several years even though the blood counts may be normal.

SUMMARY

Acquired aplastic anaemia remains a devastating and frustrating disease from which a proportion of patients still die as a result of failure of support measures. Its pathogenesis remains a mystery.

REFERENCES

Abrams SM, Degnan JJ & Vinciguerra V (1980) Marrow aplasia following topical application of chloramphenicol eye ointment. *Archives of Internal Medicine* **140:** 576–577.

Aksoy M, Dincol K, Erdem S, Akgun T & Dincol G (1972) Details of blood changes in 32 patients with pancytopenia associated with long-term exposure to benzene. *British Journal of Industrial Medicine* **29:** 56–61.

Aoki K, Fujiki N, Shimizu H & Ohno Y (1980) Geographic and ethnic differences of aplastic anaemia in humans. In: Najean Y (ed.) *Medullary Aplasia*, pp 79–88. New York: Masson.

Bacigalupo A, Podesta M, Mingari MD, Moretta L, Ling MTV & Marmont A (1980) Immune suppression of hematopoiesis in aplastic anaemia: activity of T-gamma lymphocytes. *Journal of Immunology* **125:** 1449–1453.

Baldwin JL, Storb R, Thomas ED & Mannik M (1977) Bone marrow transplantation in patients with gold induced marrow aplasia. *Arthritis and Rheumatism* **20:** 1043–1048.

Bodey GP, Bolivar R & Fainstein V (1982) Infectious complications in leukemic patients. *Seminars in Hematology* **19:** 193–226.

Bottiger LE & Bottiger B (1981) Incidence and cause of aplastic anaemia, hemolytic anaemia, agranulocytosis and thrombocytopenia. *Acta Medica Scaninavica* **210:** 475–479.

Camitta BM, Storb R & Thomas ED (1982) Aplastic anemia (first of two parts): pathogenesis, diagnosis, treatment and prognosis. *New England Journal of Medicine* **306:** 645–652.

Camitta BM, Rapeport JM, Parkman R & Nathan DG (1975) Selection of patients for bone marrow transplantation in severe aplastic anemia. *Blood* **45:** 355–363.

Canada AT & Burka ER (1968) Aplastic anemia after indomethacin. *New England Journal of Medicine* **278:** 743.

Champlin R, Ho W & Gale RP (1983) Antithymocyte globulin treatment in patients with aplastic anemia. *New England Journal of Medicine* **308:** 113–117.

De Renzo A, Formisano S, Rotoli B (1981) Bone marrow aplasia and thiamphenicol. *Haematologia* **66:** 98–104.

Dutcher JP, Schiffer CA, Aisner J & Wiernik PH (1981a) Long-term follow-up of patients with leukemia receiving platelet transfusions: identification of a large group of patients who do not become alloimmunized. *Blood* **58:** 1007–1011.

Dutcher JP, Schiffer CA, Adner J & Wiernik PH (1981b) Alloimmunization following platelet transfusion: the absence of a dose-response relationship. *Blood* **57:** 395–398.

Eernisse JG & Brand A (1981) Prevention of platelet refractoriness due to HLA antibodies by administration of leukocyte-poor blood components. *Experimental Hematology* **9:** 77–83.

Elfenbein GJ, Kallman CH, Tutschka PJ et al (1979) The immune system in 40 aplastic patients receiving conventional therapy. *Blood* **53:** 652–665.

Fraunfelder FT & Bagby GC Jr (1983) Ocular chloramphenicol and aplastic anemia. *New England Journal of Medicine* **308:** 1536.

Fraunfelder FT, Bagby GC & Kelly DJ (1982) Fatal aplastic anemia following topical administration of ophthalmic chloramphenicol. *American Journal of Ophthalmology* **93:** 356–360.

Frickhofen N, Heit W, Raghavachar A, Porzsolt F & Heimpe H (1986) Treatment of aplastic anemia with cyclosporin A, methyl prednisolone and antithymocyte globulin. *Klinische Wochenschrift* **64:** 1165–1170.

Gardner FH (1987) Haematological effects of benzene. *Seminars in Hematology* **10:** (in press).

Gaya H (1986) Combination therapy and monotherapy in the treatment of severe infection in the immunocompromised host. *American Journal of Medicine* **80:** 149–156.

Gordon MY & Gordon-Smith EC (1981) Bone marrow fibroblastoid colony-forming cells (F-CFC) in aplastic anaemia: colony growth and stimulation of granulocyte macrophage colony forming cells (GM-CFC). *British Journal of Haematology* **49:** 465–477.

Gordon MY & Gordon-Smith EC (1983) Bone marrow fibroblast function in relation to granulopoiesis in aplastic anaemia. *British Journal of Haematology* **53:** 483–489.

Gordon-Smith EC (1979) Clinical features in aplastic anemia. In: Heimpel H, Gordon-Smith EC, Heit W & Kubanek B (eds) *Aplastic Anemia—Pathophysiology and Approaches to Therapy*, pp 9–13. Heidelberg: Springer-Verlag.

Grob JP, Prentice HG, Hoffbrand AV et al (1987) Immune donors can protect marrow transplant recipients from severe cytomegalovirus infections. *Lancet* i: 774–776.

Haak H, Goselink HM, Veenhoff W, Pellinkhoff-Stadelmann S, Kleiverda JK & Te Velde J (1977) Acquired aplastic anemia in adults. IV Histological and CFU studies in transplanted and non-transplanted patients. *Scandinavian Journal of Haematology* **19:** 159–171.

Hahn FE & Gund PE (1975) A structural model of the chloramphenicol receptor site. In: Drews J & Hahn FE (eds) *Drug Receptor Interactions in Antimicrobial Chemotherapy*, vol. 1, pp 245–266. New York: Springer-Verlag.

Hara H, Kohsaki M, Noguchi K & Nagai K (1978) Effect of chloramphenicol on colony formation from erythrocytic precursors. *American Journal of Hematology* **5:** 123–130.

Heimpel H & Heit W (1980) Drug induced aplastic anaemia: clinical aspects. *Clinics in Haematology* **9:** 641–662.

Heimpel H, Heit W & Kern P (1976) Aplastic anaemias after phenylbutazone and oxyphenbutazone. *Blut* **33:** 208–213.

Herzig RH, Herzig GP, Bull MI et al (1975) Correction of poor platelet transfusion responses with leucocyte poor HLA-matched platelet concentrates. *Blood* **46:** 743–750.

Hows JM, Yin JL, Marsh J et al (1986) Histocompatible unrelated volunteer donors compared with HLA non-identical family donors in marrow transplantation for aplastic anemia and leukemia. *Blood* **68:** 1322–1328.

Inman WHW (1977) Study of fatal bone marrow depression with special reference to phenylbutazone and oxyphenbutazone. *British Medical Journal* i: 1500–1505.

International Agranulocytosis and Aplastic Anemia Study (1986) Risks of agranulocytosis and aplastic anemia: a first report of their relation to drug use with special reference to analgesics. *Journal of the American Medical Association* **256:** 1749–1757.

Jick H (1977) The discovery of drug induced illness. *New England Journal of Medicine* **296:** 481–485.

Kansu E & Erslev AJ (1976) Aplastic anemia with 'hot pockets'. *Scandinavian Journal of Haematology* **17:** 326–331.

Kay A (1973) Depression of bone marrow and thrombocytopenia associated with chrysotherapy. *Annals of Rheumatic Diseases* **33:** 277.

Kearsey SE & Craig IW (1981) Altered ribosomal RNA genes in mitochondrial mammalian cells with chloramphenicol resistance. *Nature* **290:** 607–608.

Keidan AJ, Tsatalas C, Cohen J et al (1986) Infective complications of aplastic anaemia. *British Journal of Haematology* **63:** 503–508.

Kelton JG & Ali AM (1973) Platelet transfusions—a critical appraisal. *Clinics in Oncology* **2:** 549–585.

Kickler TS, Beu WR, Ness PM, Drew H & Pall DB (1988) Leukocyte removal from platelet concentrates using a new leukocyte absorption filter. *Abstracts of Congress of the International Society of Blood Transfusion* (in press).

Klingemann HG, Self S, Banaji M et al (1987) Refractoriness to random platelet transfusions in patients with aplastic anaemia: a multivariant analysis from 264 cases. *British Journal of Haematology* **66:** 115–121.

Lancet (1986) Editorial. Analgesics, agranulocytosis and aplastic anaemia. A major case control study. *Lancet* **ii:** 899–900.

Lewis SM (1965) Course and prognosis in aplastic anaemia. *British Medical Journal* **i:** 1027–1030.

Lewis SM & Dacie JV (1967) The aplastic anaemia–paroxysmal haemoglobinuria syndrome. *British Journal of Haematology* **13:** 236–244.

Li FP, Alter BP & Nathan DG (1969) The mortality of acquired aplastic anemia in children. *Blood* **40:** 153–162.

Lynch RE, Williams DM, Reading JC & Cartwright GE (1975) The prognosis in aplastic anemia. *Blood* **45:** 517–528.

Mehta A, Gordon-Smith EC & Luzzatto L (1987) Mitochondrial DNA in patients with aplastic anaemia. *British Journal of Haematology* **66:** 416–417.

Meyers JD (1986) Infection in bone marrow transplant recipients. *American Journal of Medicine* **81:** 73–77.

Meyers JD, Fourney N & Thomas ED (1986) Risk factors for cytomegalovirus infection after human marrow transplantation. *Journal of Infectious Diseases* **153:** 478–488.

Nagro T & Maver AM (1969) Concordance for drug induced aplastic anaemia in identical twins. *New England Journal of Medicine* **281:** 7–11.

Neiweg HO (1973) Aplastic anemia (pan myelopathy). A review with special emphasis on the factors causing bone marrow damage. In: Girdwood RH (ed.) *Blood Disorders due to Drugs and other Agents*, pp 83–106. Amsterdam: Excerpta Medica.

Nissen C, Moser Y, Speck B & Bendy J (1983) Haemopoietic stimulators and inhibitors in aplastic anaemia serum. *British Journal of Haematology* **54:** 519–530.

Rich ML, Ritterhof RJ & Hoffman RL (1950) Fatal case of aplastic anemia following chloramphenicol (Chloromycetin) therapy. *Annals of Internal Medicine* **33:** 1459.

Rosenshein MS, Farewell VI, Price TH, Larson EB & Dale DC (1980) The cost effectiveness of therapeutic and prophylactic leukocyte transfusion. *New England Journal of Medicine* **302:** 1058–1062.

Sale GE, Rajantie J, Doney K, Appelbaum FR, Storb R & Thomas ED (1987) Does histologic grading of inflammation in bone marrow predict the response of aplastic anaemia patients to anti-thymocyte globulin? *British Journal of Haematology* **67:** 261–266.

Sanka CA, Besette JA, Furie B & Desforees JF (1987) Aplastic anemia complicating infectious mononucleosis. *Canadian Medical Association Journal* **136:** 730–731.

Schimpff SC, Young VM, Greene WH et al (1972) Origin of infection in acute non-lymphocytic leukemia: significance of hospital acquisition of potential pathogens. *Annals of Internal Medicine* **77:** 707–713.

Shahidi NT & Diamond LK (1959) Testosterone-induced remission in aplastic anemia. *American Journal of Diseases of Childhood* **98:** 293–301.

Slichter SJ (1980) Controversies in platelet transfusion therapy. *Annual Review of Medicine* **31:** 509–541.

Smadel JE & Jackson EB (1944) Chloromycetin, an antibiotic with chemotherapeutic activity in experimental and viral infections. *Science* **106:** 418–419.

Speck B, Gluckman E, Haak HL & van Rood JJ (1977) Treatment of aplastic anaemia by antilymphocyte globulin with and without allogeneic bone marrow infusion. *Lancet* **ii:** 1145–1148.

Storb R & Deeg HJ (1986) Failure of allogeneic canine marrow grafts after total body irradiation: allogeneic 'resistance' versus transfusion-induced sensitization. *Transplantation* **42:** 571–580.

Storb R, Thomas ED, Weiden PL et al (1974) Allogeneic marrow grafting for treatment of aplastic anemia. *Blood* **43:** 157–180.

Strauss RG (1983) Granulocyte transfusion therapy. *Clinics in Oncology* **2:** 635–655.

Stryckmans AA, Dumont JP, Velu T & Debusscher L (1984) Cyclosporine in refractory severe aplastic anemia. *New England Journal of Medicine* **310:** 655–656.

Sullivan R, Quesenberry PJ, Parkman R et al (1980) Aplastic anemia: lack of inhibitory effect of bone marrow lymphocytes on in vitro granulopoiesis. *Blood* **56:** 625–632.

Szklo M, Sensenbrenner L, Markowitz J, Weida S, Warm S & Linett M (1985) Incidence of aplastic anemia in metropolitan Baltimore: a population based study. *Blood* **66:** 115–119.

Te Velde J & Haak HL (1977) Aplastic anaemia. Histological investigation of methacrylate embedded bone marrow biopsy specimens: correlation with survival after conventional treatment in 15 adult patients. *British Journal of Haematology* **35:** 61–70.

Thomas ED & Storb R (1984) Acquired aplastic anemia. Progress and perplexity. *Blood* **64:** 325–328.

Van Saene HKF & Stoutenbeek CP (1987) Selective decontamination. *Journal of Antimicrobial Chemotherapy* **20:** 462–465.

Wallerstein RV, Condit DK, Kasper CK, Brown JW & Morrison FR (1969) Statewide study of chloramphenicol therapy and fatal aplastic anaemia. *Journal of the American Medical Association* **208:** 2045–2050.

Werner R, Kollak A, Nierhaus D, Schreiner G & Nierhaus KH (1975) Experiments on the binding sites and the action of some antibiotics which inhibit ribosomal functions. In: Drews J & Hahn FE (eds) *Drug Receptor Interactions in Antimicrobial Chemotherapy*, vol. 1, pp 217–234. New York: Springer-Verlag.

Wheeldon LW & Lehninger AL (1966) Energy-linked synthesis and decay of membrane proteins in isolated rat liver mitochondria. *Biochemistry* **5:** 3533–3545.

Wijna L, Snijder JAM & Niewig HO (1966) Acetylsalicylic acid as a cause of pancytopenia from bone marrow damage. *Lancet* **ii:** 768–770.

Williams DM, Lynch R & Cartwright GE (1973) Drug induced aplastic anemia. *Seminars in Hematology* **10:** 195–223.

Young NS, Issara Grasil S, Chieh CW & Takaku F (1986) Annotation: aplastic anaemia in the Orient. *British Journal of Haematology* **62:** 1–6.

Yunis AA, Miller AM, Salem Z & Arimura GU (1980) Chloramphenicol toxicity: pathogenetic mechanisms and the role of p-N0 sub 2 in aplastic anaemia. *Clinics in Toxicology* **17:** 354–373.

Zoumbos NC, Gascon P, Djeu JY & Young NS (1985) Circulating activated suppressor T lymphocytes in aplastic anemia. *New England Journal of Medicine* **312:** 257–265.

2

Treatment of severe aplastic anaemia

A. BACIGALUPO

The major aim of treatment of patients with aplastic anaemia is to improve the peripheral blood counts so that the patient becomes independent of transfusions and is not at risk from opportunistic infection. The two main approaches currently are allogeneic bone marrow transplantation or immunosuppressive treatment with antilymphocyte globulin (ALG). In both cases a relatively long period of intensive supportive care is necessary to keep the patient alive until self-sustaining peripheral counts are obtained, which implies that patients with aplastic anaemia should be treated mainly at transplant centres by physicians experienced in transplantation as well as in the prolonged use of corticosteroids, anabolic agents and high-quality long-term haematological support. Treatment of severe aplastic anaemia can often be quite frustrating because of slow recovery, relapses, sudden worsening of the disease or long-term complications of bone marrow transplantation. Thus both the patient and the physician should be aware that normalization of peripheral blood counts may be achieved but at a high cost in terms of personal involvement.

BONE MARROW TRANSPLANTATION

European Bone Marrow Transplant (EBMT) group results 1970–1986

Table 1 outlines the clinical data of 1090 patients reported to the EBMT

Table 1. Clinical data of 1090 severe aplastic anaemia patients reported to the EBMT registry.

	Syngeneic	HLA-identical	HLA-mismatched	Immunosuppression
Number	10	520	45	515
Age (mean)	28±8	19±13	18±12	27±17
Sex (M/F)	6/4	316/183*	26/19	259/246
Race (Caucasian Y/N)	10/0	400/120	26/19	468/52
Aetiology (Idiopathic Y/N)	8/2	353/167	23/22	349/166
Year of transfusion (1980)	3/7	239/281	12/33	187/328
Granulocyte (mean ± SD)	490±190	390±710	120±165	470±800
Platelets (mean ± SD)	21±3	17±33	12±8	16±22
Alive/dead	10/0	282/238	11/34	325/190
Follow-up—surviving patients	1162±563	1571±1085	1359±564	1103±865
Follow-up—patients dead	—	145±234	102±228	240±367

* The sex of 21 patients was not stated.

registry, including both transplanted patients and those given immunosuppression.

A total of 441 patients were treated between 1970 and 1980 and 649 between 1981 and 1986. The majority were transplanted from human leukocyte antigen (HLA)-identical sibling or received immunosuppression. A small minority received a syngeneic graft, or a transplant from a donor other than an HLA-matched sibling. All of these patients had a severe disease according to current clinical criteria (Camitta et al, 1983) as indicated by granulocyte and platelet counts at the time of treatment.

Survival curves of the four different categories of patients are given in Figure 1. All 10 patients receiving a syngeneic graft survived, although 5 of them had to be grafted twice, and their quality of life is excellent. In contrast, 45 patients receiving marrow transplants from donors other than HLA-identical siblings had an overall 23% survival rate. As will be discussed later, the use of phenotypically matched donors improves survival to over 40%.

Bone marrow transplantation and immunosuppression produce a superimposable long-term survival of 52%. The two curves are however not identical. Transplant patients show a greater mortality in the first year with

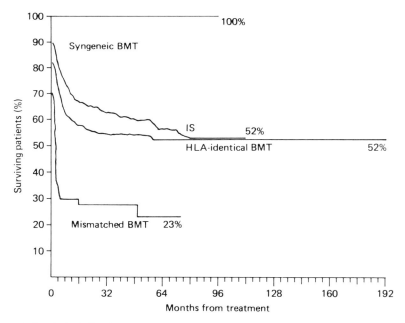

Figure 1. Survival of all patients according to treatment given: syngeneic transplants (syngeneic BMT); immunosuppression (IS), transplants from an HLA matched sibling (HLA-identical BMT), and transplants from donors other than HLA matched siblings (mismatched BMT). All recipients of a syngeneic graft survive. IS and HLA identical transplants both offer a 52% chance of long term survival. Mismatched grafts continue to be a difficult problem and produce poor results.

very few deaths beyond 24 months. The last death in this group occurred 61 months after bone marrow transplantation in a 19-year-old male transplanted in 1976; the cause was chronic graft versus host disease (GvHD) and infection. Immunosuppression-treated patients show a constant risk of death of approximately 6%/year in the second, third and fourth year: the last death occurred 69 months after immunosuppression in a 22-year-old female treated in 1977; the cause was an accident.

The overall analysis outlines the general trend for survival following different forms of treatment, but does not allow dissection of important prognostic factors. Therefore these survival curves should be interpeted with some caution and single issues will be discussed separately.

HLA TYPING

Ideally every patient with severe aplastic anaemia should be HLA-typed for three reasons—possible transplant procedures, platelet support and research purposes. Although patients over 50 years of age do not qualify for transplant procedures, they may nevertheless benefit from appropriate platelet support in case of refractoriness and may also contribute to our understanding of the association of HLA and aplasia (Bortin et al, 1981).

HLA-typing is mandatory in patients less than 40 years old with a sibling. It is also indicated in patients under 30 years of age in the absence of a sibling for possible search of an unrelated marrow donor.

IDENTICAL TWINS

One debated issue is whether patients given a syngeneic graft should be prepared with cyclophosphamide. Although the simple infusion of syngeneic marrow leads to haemopoietic reconstitution in a number of patients, approximately half fail to engraft and need to be prepared with high-dose cyclophosphamide (Appelbaum, 1980; Gale, 1981). This has been confirmed in the EBMT material: 5/10 patients were successfully regrafted after preparation with cyclophosphamide with ($n = 2$) or without ($n = 3$) buffy coat.

Initially perhaps marrow may be infused without conditioning in some cases, but it may be wise to use cyclophosphamide in most patients, especially if in poor clinical condition: time is an essential factor and there may not be time for two grafts.

Interestingly, two patients aged 62 and 69 have been successfully grafted from an identical twin after conditioning with high-dose (100–200 mg/kg) cyclophosphamide (Laffan et al, 1987). This suggests that the limitation for marrow transplantation in the elderly patient is not chemotherapy but GvHD.

HLA-IDENTICAL BONE MARROW TRANSPLANTATION

A vast experience has been accumulating on the use of HLA-identical sibling marrow transplants in severe aplastic anaemia (Storb et al, 1984; Gluckman, 1987). Survival in the range of 40% was obtained in the 1970s, especially for transfused patients (Storb et al, 1984); rejection was the main problem in almost half of the patients. This complication has been largely overcome by four separate approaches:

1. Early transplantation in untransfused patients.
2. Modified conditioning regimens including irradiation and/or various cytotoxic agents.
3. Infusion of viable donor peripheral blood cells (buffy coat) to the recipient after bone marrow transplantation.
4. The use of cyclosporin.

The result has been an improvement in survival rates to over 60%. Long-term survival in excess of 10 years is now being reported and many of these patients can be considered to be cured from the disease.

Age limit for bone marrow transplantation in aplasia

Results are clearly age-dependent, and young patients do better than older patients. However, the question is where to draw the line. A convenient cut-off point is 20 years of age since an advantage can be seen for patients younger than 20 (65% survival) compared with older patients (56%). There is no difference between patients aged 21–30 compared with patients aged 31–55 (both 56% survival; (Bacigalupo et al, 1986). Given these results, patients under 20 should be considered 'young' and patients over 20 'old'. Any therapeutic decision following diagnosis should take into account the age of the patient.

Transfusion before bone marrow transplantation

The results of bone marrow transplantation in untransfused patients are impressive—81% survive at 10 years (Storb et al, 1984) compared to the 46% survival rate of transfused patients. This is mainly due to a lower incidence of rejection in the untransfused (4/43 = 10%) compared to the transfused patients (29/93 = 33%) as predicted by the animal model (Storb et al, 1983). Young patients with severe aplastic anaemia who have an HLA-matched donor should not be transfused more than is required to keep them in a good clinical condition whilst awaiting transplant.

However, rejection can be overcome by modifications of the conditioning regimen as outlined above and the 52% rejection rate originally seen in Europe (1970–1975) has decreased to 24% from 1976 to 1980 with the addition of other agents to the regimen (mainly procarbazine and ALG) and to 17% from 1981 to 1986 (with the use of cyclosporin and irradiation; Figure 2). Other factors may contribute to the better survival of untransfused patients, namely lack of infections, lack of haemorrhages consequent on

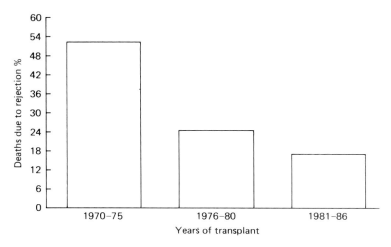

Figure 2. The impact of rejection on cumulative deaths: in the early seventies rejection represented over 50% of all deaths. This figure has dramatically dropped to 24% in 1976–80 and to 17% in 1981–86.

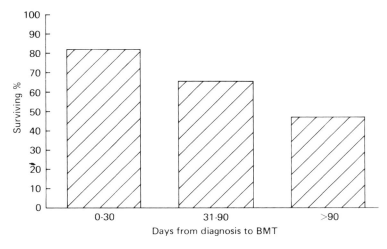

Figure 3. Effect of time from diagnosis to transplant on outcome: survival is high for patients grafted within 30 days from diagnosis. It declines thereafter for patients grafted between 31–90 days and beyond 90 days from diagnosis.

early transplantation. In keeping with this suggestion, in a recent EBMT analysis, the survival of patients grafted within 30 days ($n = 19$), between 30 and 90 days ($n = 76$) and beyond 90 days ($n = 101$) from diagnosis was respectively 82, 66 and 47% (author's unpublished observations; Figure 3). Patients treated initially with bone marrow transplantation showed higher survival rates (71%) than patients given androgen with or without steroids (47%) or immunosuppression (49%) before bone marrow transplantation (author's unpublished observations).

Thus, at present, the risks of haemorrhage and severe anaemia should be carefully considered for each patient and blood products from unrelated donors should be given if indicated. Androgens and steroids should not be used before bone marrow transplantation and the patient should be referred early to a transplant centre.

Immunosuppression with cyclophosphamide

Cyclophosphamide 200 mg/kg, administered over a period of 4 consecutive days, was initially devised as a conditioning regimen by Santos (1967). The Seattle team has shown that cyclophosphamide, together with methotrexate for GvHD prophylaxis, is an adequate conditioning regimen for untransfused but not for transfused patients (Storb et al, 1984). Cyclophosphamide given with cyclosporin as GvHD prophylaxis is an acceptable form of preparation for all patients (Hows et al, 1982). Thus the preparative regimen has to be considered in association with GvHD prophylaxis.

Given these premises, five main conditioning regimens have been used in Europe over the past years: cyclophosphamide alone, $n = 139$; cyclophosphamide + buffy coat cells, $n = 79$; cyclophosphamide + total body irradiation, $n = 33$; cyclophosphamide + total lymphoid irradiation, $n = 35$; cyclophosphamide + thoracoabdominal irradiation, $n = 114$. The results

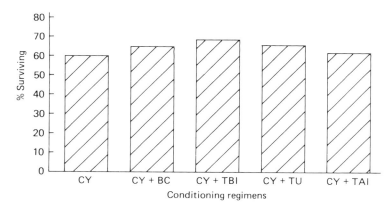

Figure 4. Effect of conditioning regimen on survival: no significant differences emerge when comparing five major conditioning regimens in patients transplanted between 1981 and 1986. CY = cyclophosphamide; CY + BC = CY and donor buffy coat post-transplant; CY + TBI = CY+ total body irradiation; CY+TU = cyclophosphamide + total lymphoid irradiation; CY+TAI = cyclophosphamide + thoraco abdominal irradiation.

obtained with these protocols are on the whole similar in terms of survival (Figure 4).

Although these data should be interpreted with caution, it seems at present that the use of irradiation does not add significantly to the survival of severe aplastic anaemia patients. It also does not produce the poor results reported by others (Storb et al, 1984). Given the possible toxic long-term effects of irradiation, it would probably be wise to reserve the combined use of cyclophosphamide and irradiation for patients sensitized to their donors through family transfusions prior to bone marrow transplantation, or for programmes involving T-cell depletion.

Influence of infused marrow cell dose

The mean cell dose received by surviving patients is 3.7 ± 1.8 compared with 3.3 ± 1.5 for patients who died (EBMT, unpublished observations). From a slightly different angle the survival of patients receiving $0.9-1.9 \times 10^8$ cells/kg ($n = 17$) is 41% and increases to 54% for patients receiving $2-3.9 \times 10^8$ cells/kg ($n = 209$) and to 60% for patients given over 4×10^8 cells/kg ($n = 184$; Figure 5). Thus, a definite beneficial effect of a high cell dose is seen in these patients, warranting efforts during marrow harvest to obtain the largest possible number of cells.

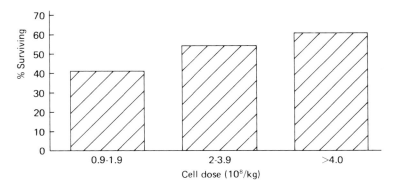

Figure 5. Effect on survival of different marrow cell doses: better results are seen for patients receiving higher doses of marrow, compared to patients receiving lower doses.

Cyclosporin versus methotrexate for GvHD prophylaxis

A report of the EBMT has shown that patients given cyclosporin have a significant survival advantage (67%) over patients given methotrexate (53%; $p = 0.001$) (Bacigalupo et al, 1986). Interestingly, this is not due to a reduced incidence and mortality of GvHD, which proved to be identical in both arms, but rather to a reduction in infections and lung complications. A recent study from Seattle has shown an advantage, both in terms of GvHD prophylaxis and survival, for patients randomized to receive cyclosporin plus methotrexate compared with patients given methotrexate alone (Storb et al, 1987). Since cyclosporin is superior in the European experience to methotrexate, the question is whether the association of cyclosporin with methotrexate is superior to cyclosporin alone. Until that is solved it would probably be wise to use cyclosporin for all patients with severe aplastic anaemia undergoing an HLA-identical sibling transplant.

T-cell depletion

There are very few reports on T-cell depletion in aplastic anaemia; the largest study is reported from Jerusalem (Or et al, 1987). Eleven patients were prepared with cyclophosphamide, high-dose TLI (1800 rad) and infused with marrow treated with Campath 1. There were two failures to achieve sustained engraftment, but nine patients survived without GvHD. The number is small and the follow-up too short to say whether T-cell depletion will improve survival overall. It should be said that survival has not improved with T-cell depletion in patients with leukaemia, and problems with chimerism and relapse continue to be of concern. It would seem that aplastic anaemia, the one disease showing a considerable incidence of graft rejection, would not be the first choice for a programme of T-cell depletion and the inclusion of T-cell depletion cannot presently be recommended for routine grafts in aplasia, and should be restricted to centres with an active on-going T-cell depletion programme.

Causes of failure

Figures 6 and 7 show the proportion of patients surviving and the causes of death in two separate periods of time: 1970–1980 and 1981–1986. An increase in survival from 43 to 63% can be seen associated with a significant reduction in deaths due to rejection (from 22 to 10%), GvHD (from 15 to 5%) and infections (from 11 to 5%).

Second marrow transplants

Thirty-seven patients received a second bone marrow transplant in the EBMT series: nine survived (24%) and 28 died. Half of the patients died of graft rejection (rejection represented 64% of all deaths); GvHD ($n = 7$) and interstitial pneumonia were the other main causes (Figure 8). A more recent analysis of second grafts in aplastic anaemia from Seattle has produced a more encouraging success rate of 40% (Storb et al, 1987b).

BONE MARROW TRANSPLANTS FROM DONORS OTHER THAN GENOTYPIC IDENTICAL SIBLINGS

The small number of such transplants performed over the past 10 years is an indication of the difficulties encountered in the selection of suitable donors

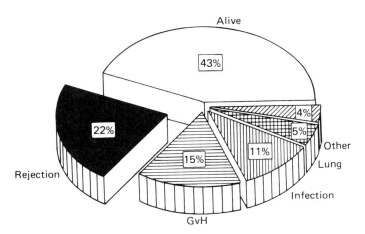

Figure 6. Causes of death in HLA identical grafts 1970–1980: rejection is the first cause of death, followed by GvH and lung toxicity.

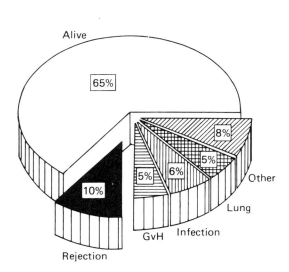

Figure 7. Causes of death in HLA identical grafts 1981–1986: a major reduction in rejection mortality is seen with an improvement of crude survival to 65%.

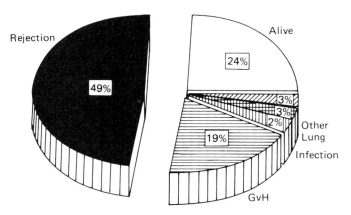

Figure 8. Causes of failure in recipients of second marrow transplants. The major cause of death is graft rejection, but lung complications and infections are also a problem.

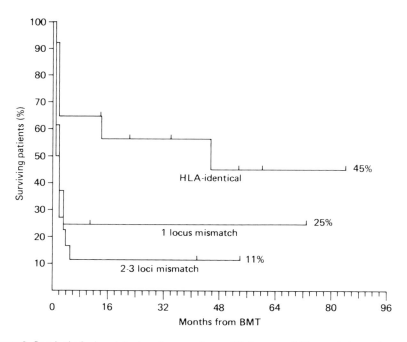

Figure 9. Survival of mismatched grafts according to HLA compatibility: recipients of marrow from phenotypic matched (HLA A, B, DR *and* MLR matched), but not genotypic matched (parents or unrelated) grafts showed best survival (45%). Mismatch for one or more loci produces poor results.

and in the transplant procedures. In Seattle 17 patients have been grafted from donors other than HLA-identical siblings: two survived for 1731 and 2203 days after the transplant; nine died of rejection and six of GvHD (Storb et al, 1984). The two survivors received a phenotypically identical marrow. Forty-five patients reported to the EBMT registry have recently been analysed (Gordon Smith et al, 1987). In this series survival could be predicted by the degree of HLA compatibility: 45% for phenotypically identical grafts, 25% for grafts mismatched at one and 11% at more than one locus (Figure 9). The problem is that HLA phenotypic identity is rare in the family outside siblings, and it is necessary to refer to unrelated donor panels.

Two successful unrelated grafts have been reported from London (Gordon Smith et al, 1982). Of the 45 EBMT patients, 11 received an unrelated graft, six of which were HLA-identical (Table 2) and of these two survive. Five were mismatched at one or more loci and none survived. Sustained engraftment without lethal GvHD can be achieved following

Table 2. HLA compatibility and donor–recipient relationship.

	Total	Alive	Dead
Donors			
Siblings	6	1	5
Parents	29	8	21
Sons	1	0	1
Unrelated	11	3	8
Phenotypic HLA compatibility			
HLA A, B, DR; MLR identical	15	8	7
Family	9	6	3
Unrelated	6	2	4
One locus mismatch	9	3	6
Family	7	3	4
Unrelated	2	0	2
Two or three loci mismatched	17	1	16
DR, MLR unknown	5	0	5

unrelated grafts but probably only in the presence of HLA phenotypic identity.

As shown in Table 2, 3/9 recipients of one locus mismatched family graft are surviving, which is a worse survival rate than in matched family donors (6/9 survivors) but comparable to unrelated matched donors (2/6 survivors). It appears that a one locus mismatched family donor is not worse than a matched unrelated donor. Two loci mismatched donors should probably not be considered at present, because of very poor results.

Given that HLA A,B,DR and MLR-matched unrelated individuals would be suitable donors for patients with severe aplastic anaemia, the problem is then their selection. The Nolan Foundation in London has recently expanded its files to 150 000 individuals but this number is probably still insufficient to find a matched donor for most patients. An international effort is clearly necessary and for this purpose the EBMT Immunology Working Party is currently organizing a European database of HLA-typed individuals.

Conditioning regimens for mismatched grafts

There is an indication from the EBMT analysis that the addition of irradiation is beneficial: survival of patients receiving cyclophosphamide together with total body or lymphoid irradiation is 31% compared to 15% for patients given cyclophosphamide alone.

T-cell depletion did not confer any advantage over methotrexate or cyclosporin; the latter ($n = 21$; survival 34%) appeared superior to both methotrexate ($n = 9$; survival 11%), and to the association of cyclosporin with marrow T-cell depletion ($n = 13$; survival 14%).

Causes of failure

The main causes of death in these patients were graft rejection ($n = 15$), GvHD ($n = 13$), pneumonitis ($n = 5$) and infections ($n = 1$). Twelve patients are alive 16–84 months after bone marrow transplantation.

IMMUNOSUPPRESSION

The use of ALG for the treatment of aplastic anaemia has proceeded through several phases. It was initially introduced by the Paris group as a 'safe' conditioning regimen before marrow infusion (Mathé, 1970) and was then used, mainly without marrow, in a small number of European centres (Speck et al, 1977). These data were then reproduced by a number of institutions (Gluckman et al, 1978; Doney et al, 1981; Jansen et al, 1982; Champlin et al, 1983; Marmont et al, 1983; Young and Speck, 1984) and ALG has now become an accepted form of treatment for aplastic anaemia. Unfortunately we know little about how ALG works or why it induces haematological reconstitution. This, associated with the lack of a definite progress in the understanding of the pathogenesis of the disease, explains why response rates to ALG (50–60%) have not improved over the past 15 years.

One thing we can do at present is to analyse these patients and our treatment schedules in order to identify prognostic factors.

Criteria for response

The degree of haematological reconstitution and the time when it occurs after ALG treatment may vary considerably from one patient to another. The EBMT group has chosen to classify as complete responders all patients not requiring blood transfusions and achieving a granulocyte count of at least $2 \times 10^9/l$ and platelet count of at least $100 \times 10^9/l$. Partial responders are transfusion-independent but do not achieve $2 \times 10^9/l$ granulocytes or $100 \times 10^9/l$ platelets. Refractory patients show no improvement.

Types of ALG

Although there have been discussions on the efficacy of different ALG preparations, results are on the whole quite comparable using different preparations (Young and Speck, 1984). In an EBMT study the two ALG brands most widely used in Europe (French: Mérieux Lymphoglobulin; Swiss: Berna Lymphoser) gave comparable results: the survival rate was 59% for 128 patients given Mérieux ALG and 64% for 136 patients receiving the Swiss ALG (Bacigalupo et al, 1986).

Addition of prednisolone

There have been no prospective controlled studies carried out to answer the question whether the addition of corticosteroids aids recovery, but in a retrospective analysis ALG and corticosteroids were not superior to ALG alone (Young and Speck, 1984). In an EBMT study low-dose prednisolone (5 mg/kg/day) plus ALG was comparable in terms of survival to high-dose prednisolone (20 mg/kg/day) together with ALG. The addition of corti-costeroids reduces the side-effects of ALG treatment (Bacigalupo et al, 1986).

Addition of androgens

One prospective study from the University of California at Los Angeles failed to show a beneficial effect of androgens given in association with ALG (Champlin et al, 1985), although the number of patients was small and the follow-up short. A second study from Frankfurt (Kaltwasser, 1987) showed an improvement in response rates (73 versus 31%) and in survival (87 versus 42%) for patients given androgens compared with patients not given androgens. A retrospective analysis of the EBMT group also showed an advantage for patients given androgens in association with ALG and pred-nisolone compared with patients receiving ALG and prednisolone without androgens (77 versus 45%; Bacigalupo et al, 1986). A prospective rando-mized trial is currently being carried out within the EBMT aplastic anaemia working party. Until the results of this study are available the usefulness of androgens should be weighed against the side-effects of their prolonged use.

Identification of responders to ALG before treatment

In vitro assays shown to correlate with clinical responses (Torok Storb, 1984; Bacigalupo et al, 1985) are difficult to perform at diagnosis in most patients because of the aplasia and the consequent very small number of cells obtained from the marrow. A second way to identify responders is to analyse clinical data of the patients at presentation. Favourable prognostic factors are a granulocyte count greater than $0.2 \times 10^9/l$, lack of infections and/or haemorrhage, older age (over 20 years), no previous treatment, drug-induced aplasia and male sex (Bacigalupo et al, 1986).

Thus young patients (less than 20 years) with very severe aplastic anaemia (granulocytes less than 0.2×10^9/l and infections or haemorrhage) seem to have the worst prognosis if treated with ALG. It is in this group of patients that identification of a suitable family or unrelated donor should be considered.

Treatment for non-responders

Further treatment depends on the age of the patient and the severity of the aplasia in the absence of an identical sibling. A second course of ALG often from a different source is effective in approximately 20% of cases (Marmont et al, 1983). This poor outlook is better than incompatible transplants unless a phenotypically identical donor is identified. Optimal haematological support with single donor platelets, possibly HLA-typed, leukocyte-poor red blood cells and appropriate antibiotic therapy will keep the patient in the best possible clinical conditions to allow recovery; some patients recover very slowly over 2 or more years.

Causes of death

Overall mortality has been reduced over the past years from 49 to 30%, but the two main causes of failure remain haemorrhage and infection.

BONE MARROW TRANSPLANTATION COMPARED WITH IMMUNOSUPPRESSION

It is not easy to select prospectively patients for bone marrow transplantation or immunosuppression other than on the basis of age and family composition. However subgroups of patients may be identified in which one treatment is superior to the other. A recent EBMT analysis suggests that bone marrow transplantation is superior to immunosuppression in patients with granulocytes less than 0.2×10^9/l (64 versus 45%; Figure 10), in patients infected (65 versus 45%) or with haemorrhages (55 versus 40%) at the time of treatment and in patients under 20 years of age (66 versus 56%; Figure 11). Immunosuppression is superior to bone marrow transplantation in patients with 0.2–0.5×10^9/l granulocytes (73 versus 59%), with over 0.5×10^9/l granulocytes (72 versus 67%), in patients not infected (68 versus 60%) or without haemorrhages (77 versus 69%) and in patients over 20 years of age (72 versus 59%; Figure 11). Survival (bone marrow transplant: immunosuppression) is not different when patients are stratified for sex (males 59:62%; females 67:60%), aetiology of the aplasia (idiopathic 57: 60%; posthepatitis 55:49%; drug-induced 82:70%), previous therapy (no 66:64%; yes 47:57%), and time from diagnosis to treatment (0–30 days: 82:66%; 31–90 days: 61:58%; over 90 days: 52:58%).

Therefore the treatment of choice for young patients with very severe aplastic anaemia is an HLA-identical bone marrow transplantation, whereas in patients over 20 years of age with moderately severe aplasia

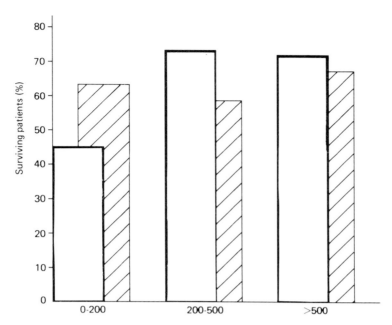

Figure 10. Effect of granulocyte (PMN) level at treatment on survival in patients receiving a graft (BMT) (▨) or immunosuppression (IS) (□) in 1981–1986. Transplantation offers an advantage over IS for patients with $<0.2 \times 10^9/l$ PMN. The opposite is true for patients with $>0.2 \times 10^9/l$ PMN.

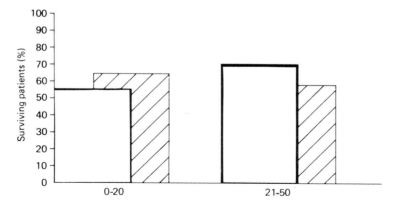

Figure 11. Effect of age on survival in patients receiving a graft (BMT) (▨) or immuno-suppression (IS) (□) in 1981–1986. An advantage for BMT patients is seen under the age of 20. The opposite is true for patients between 21 and 50.

immunosuppression produces better results. In all other groups both treatments are comparable.

Acknowledgements

This work was supported by: Associazione Italiana per la Ricerca sul Cancro (AIRC), Milan; the European Group for Bone Marrow Transplantation (EBMT); the Leukaemia Research Fund, UK; Consiglio Nazionale delle Richerche (CNR), Rome (CT 83.00870.96); Associazione Italiano contro la Leucemia (AIL), Genova.

Collection and analysis of data from the EBMT group would not have been possible without the work of Maria Teresa Van Lint and Marina Congiu.

REFERENCES

Appelbaum FR (1980) Treatment of aplastic anemia by bone marrow transplantation in identical twins. *Blood* **55**: 1033–1039.

Bacigalupo A, Podesta M, Frassoni F et al (1985) In vitro tests in severe aplastic anemia (SAA): a prospective study in 46 patients treated with immunosuppression. *British Journal of Haematology* **59**: 611–615.

Bacigalupo A, Van Lint MT, Congiu M, Pittaluga PA, Occhini D & Marmont AM (1986) Treatment of SAA in Europe 1970–1985: a report of the SAA working party. *Bone Marrow Transplantation* **1** (supplement 1): 19–21.

Bortin MM, Gale RP & Rimm AA (1981) Allogeneic bone marrow transplantation for 144 patients with severe aplastic anemia. *Journal of the American Medical Association* **245**: 1132–1139.

Camitta B, O'Reilly RJ, Sensenbrenner L et al (1983) Antithoracic duct lymphocyte globulin therapy of severe aplastic anemia. *Blood* **62**: 883–885.

Champlin R, Ho W & Gale RP (1983) Antithymocyte globulin treatment in patients with aplastic anemia: a prospective randomized trial. *New England Journal of Medicine* **308**: 113–115.

Champlin RE, Feig SA, Winston DJ, Lenarsky C & Gale RP (1985) Do androgens enhance the response to antithymocyte globulin in patients with aplastic anemia? A prospective randomized trial. *Blood* **66**: 184–188.

Doney KC, Weiden PL, Buckner CD, Storb R & Thomas ED (1981) Treatment of severe aplastic anemia using antithymocyte globulin with or without an infusion of HLA haploidentical marrow. *Experimental Hematology* **9**: 829–833.

Gale RP (1981) Aplastic anemia: biology and treatment. *Annals of Internal Medicine* **95**: 477–496.

Gluckman E (1987) Current status of bone marrow transplantation for severe aplastic anemia: a preliminary report from the International Bone Marrow Transplant Registry. *Transplant Proceedings* **XIX**: 2597–2599.

Gluckman E, Devergie A, Faille A, Barrett AJ, Bonneau M & Bernard J (1978) Treatment of severe aplastic anemia with antilymphocyte globulin and androgens. *Experimental Hematology* **6**: 679–687.

Gordon Smith EC, Fairhead SM & Chipping PM (1982) Bone marrow transplantation for severe aplastic anemia using histocompatible unrelated volunteer donors. *British Medical Journal* **285**: 835–837.

Gordon Smith EC, Hows J, Bacigalupo A et al (1987) Bone marrow transplantation for severe aplastic anemia (SAA) from donors other than HLA identical siblings: a report of the EBMT working party. *Bone Marrow Transplantation* **2** (supplement 1): 100.

Hows J, Palmer S & Gordon Smith EC (1982) Use of cyclosporin A in allogeneic bone marrow transplantation for severe aplastic anemia. *Transplantation* **33**: 382–386.

Jansen J, Zwaan F & Haak HL (1982) Antithymocyte globulin treatment for aplastic anemia. *Scandinavian Journal of Hematology* **28**: 341–351.

Kaltwasser JP, Dix U, Schalk KP & Vogt H (1988) Effect of androgens on the response to antithymocyte globulin in patients with aplastic anaemia. *European Journal of Haematology* **40**: 111–118.

Laffan M, Durrent S, Harhalakis N, Economou K, Hows JM & Gordon Smith EC (1987) Bone marrow transplantation in the elderly. *Bone Marrow Transplantation* **2** (supplement 1): 105.

Marmont AM, Bacigalupo A, Van Lint MT et al (1983) Treatment of severe aplastic anemia with sequential immunosuppression. *Experimental Hematology* **11**: 856–865.

Mathé G (1970) Bone marrow graft in man after conditioning with antithymocyte serum. *British Medical Journal* **2**: 131–136.

Or R, Naparstek E, Weiss L et al (1987) BMT in severe aplastic anemia (SAA) using HLA identical allografts T cell depleted by Campath 1. *Bone Marrow Transplantation* **2** (supplement 1): 119.

Santos GW (1967) Induction of specific tolerance to soluble and particulate antigens in man and tissue allografts in mice with cyclophosphamide. *Experimental Hematology* **14**: 32–34.

Speck B, Gluckman E, Haak HL & Van Rood JJ (1977) Treatment of aplastic anemia by antithymocyte globulin with and without allogeneic bone marrow infusions. *Lancet* **ii**: 1145–1147.

Storb R, Prentice RL, Thomas ED et al (1983) Factors associated with graft rejection after HLA identical marrow transplantation. *British Journal of Haematology* **55**: 573–585.

Storb R, Thomas ED, Appelbaum FR et al (1984) Marrow transplantation for severe aplastic anemia: the Seattle experience. In Young NS, Levine A & Humphries RK (eds) *Aplastic Anemia: Stem Cell Biology and Advances in Treatment*, pp 297–313. New York: Alan R. Liss.

Storb R, Deeg HJ, Farewell V et al (1987) Marrow transplantation for severe aplastic anemia: methotrexate alone compared with a combination of methotrexate and cyclosporin for prevention of acute graft versus host disease. *Blood* **68**: 119–125.

Storb R, Weiden PL, Sullivan KM et al (1987) Second marrow transplants in patients with aplastic anemia rejecting their first graft: use of a conditioning regimen including cyclophosphamide and antilymphocytic globulin. *Blood* **70**: 116–121.

Torok Storb BJ (1984) T cell effects on in vitro erythropoiesis: immune regulation and immune reactivity. In Young NS, Levine A & Humphries RK (eds) *Aplastic Anemia: Stem Cell Biology and Advances in Treatment*, pp 163–172. New York: Alan R. Liss.

Young N & Speck B (1984) Antithymocyte and antilymphocyte globulins: clinical trials and mechanism of action. In Young NS, Levine A & Humphries RK (eds) *Aplastic Anemia: Stem Cell Biology and Advances in Treatment*, pp 221–226. New York: Alan R. Liss.

Centers contributing patients to the EBMT Registry: Barcellona, A Granena, Basel, B Speck, Bergamo, T Barbui, Birmingham, Franklin, Bologna, P Ricci, Bolzano, P Coser, Bordeaux, J Reiffers, Budapest, A Poros, Charing Cross, HP Davis, Copenhagen, P Ernst, Cuneo, G Gallamini, Dublin, S McCann, Edinburgh, AC Parker, Eduard Herriot, H Fiere, Essen, U Schaefer, Firenze, A Bosi, Gaslini, PG Mori, Grenoble, Michalet, Hammersmith, J Hows, Helsinki, MA Siimes, Hotel Dieux, Baunelon, Huddinge, O Ringden, Jerusalem, S Slavin, Insbruck, D Niederwieser, Leiden Adults, M de Planque, Leiden Pediatrics, J Vossen, Lovanio, GJK Tricot, Marseille, Maraninchi, Modena, Silingardi, Monza, C Uderzo, Nancy, T Bordigoni, Nice, Gratecos, Palermo, M Lo Curto, Pavia, E Ascari, Pavia, F Porta, Pesaro, P Polchi, Pescara, P Di Bartolomeo, Rom, W Arcese, Royal Free, G Prentice, Royal Marsden, R Powles, Saint Louis, E Gluckman, Salpetrier, Binet, San Giovanni Rotondo, M Carotenuto, Saint Etienne, Freycon, San Pau, Brunet, Torino, L Resegotti, Torino, M Aglietta, Torino, P Saracco, Tubingen, Ostendorf, Turku, A Toivanen, Ulm, H Heimpel, Vicenza, T Chisesi, Vienna, W Hinterbeger, Westminster, J Barrett, Zurich, J Gmur.

3

Pathophysiology of aplastic anaemia

CATHERINE NISSEN-DRUEY

Despite 20 years of research the underlying cause of aplastic anaemia remains unknown. However, advances in clinical and experimental haematology have contributed significantly to insight into the pathophysiological mechanisms involved. In this chapter the findings that have improved our understanding of the disease will be reviewed and a new concept which unites apparently controversial ideas will be presented.

Before the development of supportive care and new antibiotics the severe form of aplastic anaemia was almost invariably rapidly fatal. Aplastic anaemia was then considered to be a variant of acute leukaemia presenting with marrow hypoplasia. Patients can now be kept alive without specific treatment for several years and aplastic anaemia is currently regarded as a more benign disease than acute leukaemia.

ASSOCIATION WITH DRUGS, CHEMICALS AND VIRUSES

When the association between aplastic anaemia and exposure to certain drugs, chemicals and viruses became evident, these agents were thought to be the primary cause of the disease. However, since only a small minority of exposed individuals develop aplastic anaemia, these agents should rather be thought of as risk factors or 'triggers' which induce bone marrow failure only in certain susceptible individuals. The classification into drug or virus-induced aplastic anaemia is somewhat arbitrary. As will be shown, drugs and viruses probably play a similar role in the pathophysiology of aplastic anaemia.

Drugs and chemicals

A list of agents that have no dose-dependent cytotoxicity, but are occasionally associated with marrow hypoplasia, is given in Table 1. It shows that virtually any drug may be involved. For some compounds the association is strong. For frequently used drugs, such as analgesics, the risk of developing aplastic anaemia after exposure is small but it is important to know if the risk is significant. In a large population study (International Agranulocytosis and

38 C. NISSEN-DRUEY

Table 1. Chemical and physical agents occasionally associated with marrow hypoplasia.

Class of compound	20 or more reported cases	Single or few reports
Antimicrobial agents	Chloramphenicol	Streptomycin, penicillin, methicillin
	Organic arsenicals	Oxytetracycline, chlortetracycline, sulphonamides
	Quinacrine	Sulphisoxazole, sulphamethoxy-pyridazine, amphotericin B
Anticonvulsants	Methylphenylethylhydantoin, Trimethadione	Phenacemide, phenurone/diphenyl-hydantoin, ethosuximide, carbamazepine
Antithyroid drugs		Carbethoxythiomethylglyoxaline, potassium perchlorate, propylthiouracil
Antidiabetic agents		Tolbutamide, chlorpropamide, carbutamide
Antihistamines		Tripelennamine
Analgesics	Phenylbutazone	Acetyl salicylic acid, indomethacin
Sedatives and tranquillizers		Meprobamate, chlorpromazine, promazine, chlordiazepoxide, mepazine, methyprylon
Insecticides		Chlorophenothane (DDT), parathion, chlordane, pentachlorophenol
Miscellaneous	Gold compounds	Acetazolamide, hair dyes, methazolamide, dinitrophenol, thiocyanate, bismuth, mercury, D-penicillamine, colloidal silver, carbon tetrachloride, solvents, cimetidine, metolazone

From Wintrobe (1981).

Aplastic Anemia Study, 1986) indomethacin was found to increase the risk from 2.2 to 10.1 per million per year; it was increased to 6.8 by exposure to diclofenac sodium and to 6.6 per million per year by butazones.

Chloramphenicol has been studied in detail as an inducer of aplastic anaemia. Its dose-dependent toxicity has been ascribed to mitochondrial damage (Yunis et al, 1980). However, the rare, dose-independent, irreversible toxicity is hardly explained by this mechanism. Lymphocytes from patients who have recovered from chloramphenicol-induced aplastic anaemia can be stimulated in vitro with the drug (Schultz et al, 1979), indicating that immune mechanisms may play a role. Low doses of chloramphenicol stimulate rather than inhibit normal haemopoietic precursor cells in vitro (Bostrom et al, 1986). These observations indicate that the drug interacts with lymphohaemopoietic cells in a primarily non-cytotoxic way. At high doses chloramphenicol is suppressive in vitro. Genetic factors appear to determine individual sensitivity, since firstly, bone marrow cells from relatives of patients with chloramphenicol-induced aplastic anaemia are more sensitive to the drug than those from normal individuals (Yunis, 1973); secondly, the sensitivity differs among mouse strains (Yunis et al, 1980), and thirdly, chloramphenicol-induced aplastic anaemia has occurred simultaneously in identical twins (Nago and Maurer, 1969). A hypothetical explanation for these findings could be that chloramphenicol becomes antigenic by interacting with certain rare human leukocyte antigen molecules (see below) and thus induces an autoimmune reaction.

Aplastic anaemia can be due to direct bone marrow toxicity, as after exposure to acetanilide. Acetanilide is cleared more slowly in susceptible individuals, although clearance is normal in patients with idiopathic aplastic anaemia (Cunningham et al, 1974). Thus, there are different pathophysiological mechanisms by which drugs and chemicals can cause or contribute to bone marrow failure.

Viruses and infection

Aplastic anaemia can occur during or early after viral hepatitis (Ajouni and Doeblin, 1974; Hagler et al, 1975; Abe and Komiya, 1978; Böttiger, 1978) or exposure to other viruses, such as the Epstein–Barr virus. Herpes simplex infection in aplastic anaemia patients frequently precedes a reduction in peripheral blood counts or frank relapse (Nissen-Druey unpublished data). Similarly, bacterial and fungal infections depress bone marrow function in aplastic anaemia patients.

Since only a minority of infected patients develop bone marrow failure, infection seems to act as a trigger rather than be the cause. Pregnancy is another known risk factor. It is conceivable that an immune imbalance of any origin can act as a trigger. Viral infections and drugs can potentiate each other as risk factors, e.g. the incidence of aplastic anaemia rises sharply after exposure to a virus and a drug, such as for example hepatitis and chloramphenicol (Hagler et al, 1975). Viruses which actually destroy haemopoietic cells resulting in bone marrow failure (Saarinen et al, 1976; Mortimer et al, 1983; Young et al, 1984) are not detectable in classical aplastic anaemia.

Since pancytopenia is a prominent feature of acquired immune deficiency syndrome (AIDS), it was postulated that a retrovirus might be involved in the pathogenesis of aplastic anaemia. In bone marrow and peripheral blood samples from 40 patients with aplastic anaemia (including acute severe disease) retroviral DNA, reverse transcriptase or specific antibodies to any of the known human retroviruses could not be detected (Mullins et al, unpublished data).

Despite these negative data, it remains an open question whether a novel virus plays a key role in the pathogenesis of aplastic anaemia.

CLINICAL OBSERVATIONS

The two main treatment modalities for aplastic anaemia are bone marrow transplantation and high-dose immunosuppression with antilymphocyte globulin. New insights were obtained from treatment results in these two groups of patients. The observation that aplastic anaemia can be cured by bone marrow transplantation suggested that the cause of aplastic anaemia is a lack of normal haemopoietic stem cells. On the other hand, autologous bone marrow reconstitution after high-dose immunosuppression would not occur if there were no normal haemopoietic cells in the apparently empty marrow. The question of whether aplastic anaemia is a disease of the 'seed' or the 'soil' has been discussed at length. There is clinical evidence to support both hypotheses. Some identical twin recipients engraft donor marrow without previous immunosuppression, whereas others require preparation. These results could be explained by either an intrinsic defect of the haemopoietic stem cells, i.e. a disease of the 'seed', or a primary defect of the 'soil' which does not allow normal marrow to engraft. Likewise, it was assumed that patients who do not respond to immunosuppressive treatment have a disease of the 'seed', whereas 'responders' have a disease of the 'soil'. Time and experience have shown that 'response' and 'non-response' are inadequate criteria. Firstly, a patient can recover many months after being considered a 'non-responder; secondly, the response rates at different treatment centres vary widely, indicating that 'response' is an inappropriate pathophysiological parameter. It is possible that all patients are potential responders, but the clinical outcome depends on which progresses faster, autologous bone marrow recovery or the disease process.

Although bone marrow function improves after immunosuppression, clinical experience teaches us that immune mechanisms are probably not the primary cause. Whereas a bone marrow graft usually cures the disease, haemopoiesis does not fully recover after immunosuppression with the exception of rare patients. Relapse occurs and transition to potentially lethal clonal haemopoietic diseases is seen more frequently after immunosuppression with increasing observation time (de Planque et al, 1987a; Tichelli et al, 1987). Thus, the disease appears to affect both 'seed' and 'soil'.

Aplastic anaemia has often been regarded as a heterogeneous disease. Clinical results indicate that this is probably not the case. Looking at patients in autologous bone marrow remission, we see no difference between those who have recovered from chloramphenicol-induced, postviral or idiopathic aplasia. The majority of patients have residual clinical signs of the disease (de Planque et al, 1987b) and all have abnormalities of haemopoiesis in vitro, including firstly, grossly reduced proliferative capacity of haemopoietic precursors (Bacigalupo et al, 1980b; Nissen et al, 1980; Torres et al, 1983; Yoshida et al, 1983; Ruvidic et al, 1985); secondly, unexplained sensitivity of precursor cells to complement (Nissen et al, 1986) and thirdly, excess production of haemopoietic growth factors by peripheral blood cells (Nissen et al, 1986a). They are equally prone to relapse and the development of clonal diseases of haemopoiesis, even years after therapy. In our experience, only patients who had aplasia after exposure to drugs other than chloramphenicol have the potential to recover autologous haemopoiesis to complete normality. This reversible type of aplasia resembles drug-induced agranulocytosis but involves all haemopoietic lineages.

IN VITRO CULTURES

Evidence for an intrinsic defect of haemopoietic cells

Aplastic bone marrow has a very low proliferative capacity in culture (Kern et al, 1977). The response of precursor cells to haemopoietic growth factors (including GM-CSF and IL-3) is decreased or absent. This defect does not normalize after immunosuppressive therapy (Bacigalupo et al, 1980; Nissen et al, 1980; Torres et al, 1983; Yoshida et al, 1983; Ruvidic et al, 1985). Cultures from aplastic anaemia patients resemble cultures from preleukaemia, with one exception. Macrophage or fibroblast clusters from many aplastic bone marrow grow abundantly (Figure 1) and they are sometimes surrounded by haemopoietic cells. Such clusters are sometimes—more rarely—seen in cultures from patients with preleukaemia. Cells grown from such clusters produce large amounts of haemopoietic growth factors, allowing one to speculate that the clusters represent factor-producing cells which are stimulated to produce excess growth factors in an attempt to rectify the lesion in aplastic anaemia. Intrinsic abnormalities are not restricted to

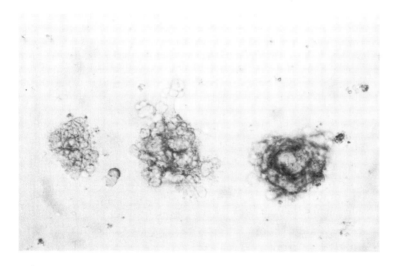

Figure 1. Macrophage or fibroblast clusters in culture of aplastic anaemia bone marrow.

haemopoietic precursors: bone marrow stroma cells from aplastic marrow also do not proliferate normally in culture (Warren et al, 1980; Wiktor-Jedrzeijczak et al, 1982; Torok-Storb, 1984; Elstner et al, 1985; Hotta et al, 1985; Juneja and Gardner, 1985) and in peripheral blood lymphocytes from aplastic anaemia patients a defect of DNA repair has been found (Morley et al, 1978; Kovacs et al, 1987). Both these abnormalities persist to a variable extent in autologous remission (Kovacs et al, unpublished data). Interestingly aplastic anaemia lymphocytes which have abnormally low DNA repair synthesis proliferate strongly on stimulation with lectins, showing that replicative DNA synthesis is normal.

The cause of these intrinsic cellular abnormalities is unknown. They resemble findings in congenital Fanconi's anaemia. In aplastic anaemia they seem to be acquired rather than congenital.

Evidence for immune mechanisms

Improvement of haemopoietic function after immunosuppressive treatment is the strongest argument for the involvement of immune mechanisms in the pathophysiology of aplastic anaemia. The observation originally stimulated the search for a specific harmful immunological agent—antibody, cytotoxic T-cell, monocyte-macrophage or lymphokine. Each has been incriminated but none has proved to be the sole cause of bone marrow failure. They will be considered separately below.

Antibodies

The target of autoaggression in aplastic anaemia is probably a multipotential haemopoietic cell with extensive proliferation capacity. Since aplastic bone marrow does not proliferate in culture normal bone marrow cells have been used as a substitute target for detection of autoimmunity in vitro. With such allogeneic coculture experiments it has been found that aplastic anaemia is not an autoimmune disease in the classical sense. Antibodies against normal precursor cells are rarely detectable in patient serum. Patient serum stimulates rather than inhibits normal as well as autologous precursor cells (Nissen et al, 1979, 1985a,b). Hence, classical aplastic anaemia is not a typical autoimmune disease, except in rare cases (Freedman et al, 1979; Fitchen and Cline, 1980). This does not rule out a role for antibody in the disease process. For instance, the IgM fraction of pretreatment serum inhibits autologous colony formation and production of haemopoietic growth factors by cells from patients in remission (Nissen et al, 1983, 1984). Since such inhibitory serum activities are counteracted by stong haemopoietic stimulators (Nissen et al, 1985a,b, 1986a) it is not surprising that they are missed when whole serum is tested for autoantibodies. It is possible that antibodies only act in co-operation with immune-competent cells to cause marrow failure.

T-lymphocytes

T-lymphocytes, mainly of the CD8 phenotype, from aplastic anaemia patients have been shown to inhibit colony formation by both allogeneic and autologous haemopoietic colony-forming cells (Kagan et al, 1976; Hoffman et al, 1977; Singer et al, 1978; Torok-Storb et al, 1978, 1980; Gorski et al, 1979; Bacigalupo et al, 1980a, 1981; Zoumbos et al, 1985a; Hanada et al, 1986). However, the phenomenon of T-cell-mediated bone marrow suppression could not be reproduced by all groups (Sullivan et al, 1980).

Many observations indicate that T-cells do not actually cause aplastic anaemia:

1. There is no overt imbalance of T-lymphocyte subsets in aplastic anaemia (Falcao et al, 1984a; Ruiz-Arguelles et al, 1984; Wang et al, 1986) except for posthepatitic aplasia in which a low CD4 : CD8 ratio has been reported (Wang et al, 1986).

PATHOPHYSIOLOGY OF APLASTIC ANAEMIA

2. Normal lymphocytes can also inhibit bone marrow function in vitro (Morris et al, 1984) and in general immunological autoreactivity is a physiological phenomenon (Claesson and Olsson, 1980).
3. Treatment of aplastic anaemia with a monoclonal pan-T-antibody does not induce remission.
4. Attempts to create autocytotoxic T-lymphocytes against bone marrow have failed (Nissen and Goulmy, unpublished data).

Even though T-cells alone do not cause aplastic anaemia, the fact that they are activated during the acute stage of the disease may be important

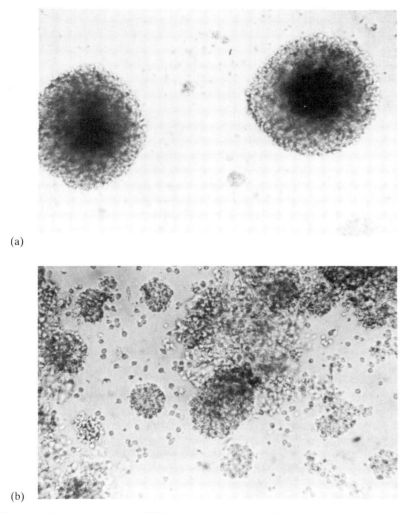

(a)

(b)

Figure 2. Growth patterns of PHA-stimulated peripheral blood lymphocytes from aplastic anaemia **(a)** on admission; **(b)** in autologous remission.

(Finlay et al, 1980; Zoumbos et al, 1984). Peripheral blood cells from untreated patients form very large spherical T-cell colonies in >80% of cases (Figure 2a). This phenomenon probably also reflects activation, since it disappears in remission (Figure 2b). In about 20% of patients, T-cell colony formation on admission is poor or absent. These patients have the most severe form of aplastic anaemia in which lymphocytes are apparently also involved in the disease process.

Monocyte-macrophages

These have been shown to inhibit autologous colony formation in culture (Nissen et al, 1980; Suda et al, 1980, 1981; Takaku et al, 1980). Again, they are unlikely to be the sole cause of marrow failure, particularly since patients with severe monocytopenia usually have very severe disease and a poor prognosis.

Lymphokines

The role of lymphokines in the pathophysiology of aplastic anaemia has been debated. The release of interleukin-2 (IL-2) by peripheral blood cells is high in about 60% of patients in the acute phase (Gascon et al, 1985; Nissen et al, 1986a) and tends to normalize in remission (Nissen et al, 1986a). However, IL-2 is unlikely to be the only cause of aplasia since lymphocytes from some patients continue to release excess IL-2 in remission. The same holds true for interferon–gamma (IF-γ). Patient cells release excess IF-γ on lectin stimulation (Mangan et al, 1985; Zoumbos et al, 1985b). IF-γ production does not correlate with the degree of bone marrow failure (Hanada et al, 1987) and its myelosuppressive activity could not be reproduced (Torok-Storb et al, 1987).

Other immune mechanisms such as circulating immune complexes (Caligaris et al, 1980) and an increased level of soluble circulating T-sheep red cell receptors (Falcao et al, 1984b) have been described in aplastic anaemia. They are further signs of immune activation.

In conclusion, the attempt to find a single causative immunological agent is inappropriate. Rather, the entire immune system is activated and probably involved in causing bone marrow damage. In addition, there is a problem with the experiments designed to demonstrate immune phenomena in aplastic anaemia, in that normal cells are taken as controls. To use cells from patients who have an activated immune system but do not develop bone marrow failure would be more interesting and approach the central problem—the nature of the antigenic stimulus in aplastic anaemia.

THE ROLE OF REGULATORY CELLS

As mentioned earlier, the haemopoietic defect in aplastic anaemia involves environmental cells. Could marrow failure result from an inadequate supply of haemopoietic growth factors? Accessory cells are involved to widely varying extents in different patients. In bone marrow stroma cultures from some patients there is abundant growth of fibroblasts which, although unable to support autologous haemopoiesis, release an excess of haemopoietic growth factors. In rare patients no fibroblast growth and thus no factor production is seen (author's unpublished data). This difference is also reflected by the varying ability of patients' peripheral blood cells to release haemopoietic growth factors. In some patients production is very low—a fact which may aggravate the disease. Low production is indeed associated with very severe disease. In some it is abnormally high (Nissen et al, 1982) but obviously not capable of correcting bone marrow failure. The primary defect is a failure in response rather than in production of growth factors. Since there is no cut off point between high and low producers, inadequate factor supply does not seem to characterize a disease entity of its own; rather it is a symptom of severe disease involving both haemopoietic and regulatory cells. The IgM fraction from patient pretreatment serum is inhibitory to haemopoietic growth factor release by autologous peripheral blood cells (Nissen et al, 1983), indicating that an antibody may be involved in the damage to environmental cells.

GENETIC FACTORS

Marrow sensitivity to chloramphenicol appears to have a genetic element. It has also been shown that aplastic anaemia of any cause is linked to certain histocompatibility antigens. An increased frequency of human leukocyte antigen DR2 in patients and increased sharing of DR antigens in their parents was found (Chapuis et al, 1986). In a small group of aplastic anaemia patients the frequency of DPw3 was highly significantly increased (Odum et al, 1987). Similar findings have been made in acute leukaemia patients and their relatives. Aplastic anaemia, although a more benign disease, does share features with acute leukaemia.

SUMMARY

No single pathophysiological phenomenon—neither the intrinsic defect of haemopoiesis nor any of the described immune effects—explains aplastic anaemia. Since the intrinsic defect is compatible with near normal haemopoietic function, as seen in autologous bone marrow reconstitution, it cannot be the cause of severe pancytopenia. On the other hand, immune mechanisms cannot be the primary cause of the disease, otherwise haemopoietic function would recover to complete normality after immunosuppressive therapy. From these observations we deduce that the intrinsic defect, a premalignant haemopoietic disorder, can either be clinically quiescent by virtue of repair mechanisms, or induce auto-reactivity of the immune system against the abnormal haemopoietic tissue, drugs, chemicals and viruses acting as non-specific triggers or amplifiers. In this sense, aplastic anaemia could be interpreted as an attempt to 'self-cure' from a variant type of preleukaemia. This means that the original concept of aplastic anaemia being a hypoplastic variant of leukaemia may be true. The fact that aplastic anaemia can present either as acute severe bone marrow failure, as chronic mild pancytopenia or as a myelodysplasia-like syndrome does not imply that the underlying pathophysiological mechanisms are basically different. Variations of the clinical course and the response to immunosuppressive treatment could be explained by variations in the balance between the primary defect and the secondary immune reaction; the co-involvement of accessory cells in the primary disease; the relative time course of the two components and the efficiency of repair mechanisms. From repeated in vitro studies in a large group of aplastic anaemia patients at various stages of disease this concept can be applied to the majority of cases, including chloramphenicol- and virus-induced aplastic anaemia. In a small proportion of patients with pancytopenia occurring after exposure to certain drugs other than cloramphenicol, aplastic anaemia is rapidly and completely reversible after withdrawal of the drug. These patients probably have truly benign aplastic anaemia and thus differ from the majority of patients who are left with a permanently fragile bone marrow once they have acquired aplastic anaemia.

REFERENCES

Abe T & Komiya M (1978) Some clinical aspects of aplastic anemia. In: *Aplastic Anemia*, pp 197–204. Tokyo: University of Tokyo.

Ajouni K & Doeblin TD (1974) The syndrome of hepatitis and aplastic anaemia. *British Journal of Haematology* 27: 345–355.

Bacigalupo A, Podestà M, Mingari MC et al (1980a) Immune suppression of hematopoiesis in aplastic anemia: activity of T-gamma-lymphocytes. *Journal of Immunology* 125: 1449–1453.

Bacigalupo A, Podesta M & Raffo MR (1980b) Lack of in vitro colony (CFU) formation and myelosuppressive activity in patients with severe aplastic anemia after autologous hematologic reconstitution. *Experimental Hematology* 8(6): 795–801.

Bacigalupo A, Podesta M, van Lint MT et al (1981) Severe aplastic anaemia: correlation of in vitro tests with clinical response to immunosuppression in 20 patients. *British Journal of Haematology* 47: 423–432.

Bostrom B, Smith K & Ramsay KC (1986) Stimulation of human committed bone marrow stem cells (CFU-GM) by cloramphenicol. *Experimental Hematology* 14: 156–161.

Böttiger IE (1978) Prevalance and etiology of aplastic anemia in Sweden. In: *Aplastic Anemia*, pp 171–180. Tokyo: University of Tokyo.

Caligaris FC, Novarino A, Camussi G & Gavosto F (1980) Immune complexes in aplastic anaemia. *British Journal of Haematology* 45: 81–87.

Chapuis B, v. Fliedner VE, Jeannet M et al (1986) Increased frequency of DR2 in patients with aplastic anaemia and increased DR-sharing in their parents. *British Journal of Haematology* 63: 51–57.

Claesson MH & Olsson L (1980) Autoreactive natural killer cells from agar cloned murine bone marrow cells. *Nature* 283: 578–580.

Cunningham JL, Leyland MJ, Delamore IW & Price EDA (1974) Acetanilide oxidation in oxidation in phenylbutazone-associated hypoplastic anaemia. *British Medical Journal* 3: 313–317.

de Planque M, Brand A, Eernisse JG et al (1987a) Quantitatively and qualitatively abnormal hematopoiesis of severe aplastic anemia (SAA) patients who have improved after antithymocyte globuline (ATG) treatment. *Bone Marrow Transplantation* 2(supplement 1): 109.

de Planque M, Kluin-Nelemans JC, v. Krieken JHJM & Zwaan FE (1987b) Leukaemia following myelodysplasia after aplastic anaemia. *Bone Marrow Transplantation* **2(supplement 1):** 110.

Elstner E, Schulze E, Ihle R, Stobbe H & Grunze S (1985) Stromal progenitor cells in bone marrow of patients with aplastic anemia. *Haematology and Blood Transfusion* **29:** 168–171.

Falcao RP, Voltarelli JC & Bottura C (1984a) T-cell subsets in patients with aplastic anemia. *Brazilian Journal of Medical and Biological Research* **17(2):** 151–156.

Falcao RP, Longo IM, Moura NC & Mendes NF (1984b) Quantification of the soluble receptor of human T-lymphocytes for sheep erythrocytes in the serum of patients with aplastic anemia. *Journal of Clinical Laboratory Immunology* **13(3):** 141–143.

Finlay JL, Ershler WB & Shahidi NT (1980) Immunologic mechanisms in aplastic anemia. *American Journal of Pediatric Hematology and Oncology* **2(3):** 223–232.

Fitchen JH & Cline MJ (1980) Serum inhibitors of myelopoiesis. *British Journal of Haematology* **44:** 7–16.

Freedman MH, Gelfand EW & Saunders EF (1979) Acquired aplastic anemia: antibody mediated hemopoietic failure. *American Journal of Hematology* **6(2):** 135–141.

Gascon P, Zoumbos NC, Scala G et al (1985) Lymphokine abnormalities in aplastic anemia: implications for the mechanism of action of antithymocyte globulin. *Blood* **65:** 407–413.

Gorski A, Rowinska D, Skopinska E & Orlowski T (1979) Circulating suppressor cells in aplastic anaemia. *Vox Sanguinis* **36:** 356–361.

Hagler L, Pastore, Bergin JJ et al (1975) Aplastic anemia following viral hepatitis: report of two fatal cases and literature review. *Medicine (Baltimore)* **54(2):** 136–164.

Hanada T, Aoki Y, Ninomiya H & Abe T (1986) T-cell mediated inhibition of haemopoiesis in aplastic anaemia: serial assay of inhibitory activities of T cells to autologous CFU-E during immunosuppressive therapy. *British Journal of Haematology* **63(1):** 69–74.

Hanada T, Yamamura H, Ehara T et al (1987) No evidence for gamma-interferon mediated inhibition by T-cells in aplastic anaemia: an observation in the course of immunosuppressive therapy. *British Journal of Haematology* **67:** 123–127.

Hoffman R, Zanjani ED & Lutton JD (1977) Suppression of erythroid colony formation by lymphocytes from patients with aplastic anaemia. *New England Journal of Medicine* **296:** 10–13.

Hotta T, Kato T, Maeda H et al (1985) Functional changes in marrow stromal cells in aplastic anaemia. *Acta Haematologica (Basel)* **74(2):** 65–69.

International Agranulocytosis and Aplastic Anemia Study (1986) Risks of agranulocytosis and aplastic anemia: a first report of their relation to drug use with special reference to analgesics. *Journal of the American Medical Association* **256:** 1749–1759.

Juneja HS & Gardner FH (1985) Functionally abnormal marrow stromal cells in aplastic anemia. *Experimental Hematology* **13(3):** 194–199.

Kagan W, Ascensao JA, Pahwa RN et al (1976) Aplastic anemia: presence in human bone marrow of cells that suppress myelopoiesis. *Proceedings of the National Academy of Sciences USA* **73:** 2890–2894.

Kern P, Heimpel H, Heit W & Kubanek B (1977) Granulocytic progenitor cells in aplastic anemia. *British Journal of Haematology* **35:** 613–623.

Kovacs E, Nissen C, Speck B & Signer E (1987) Repair of UV-induced DNA damage in aplastic anemia: changes after treatment with antilymphocyte globulin (ALG). *European Journal of Haematology* **40:** 430–436.

Mangan KF, Zidar B, Shadduck RK, Zeigler Z & Winkelstein A (1985) Interferon-induced aplasia: evidence for T-cell-mediated suppression of hematopoiesis and recovery after treatment with horse antihuman thymocyte globulin. *American Journal of Hematology* **19(4):** 401–413.

Morley A, Trainor K & Remes J (1978) Is aplastic anaemia due to an abnormality of DNA? *Lancet* **ii:** 9–11.

Morris TC, Vincent PC, Young GA et al (1984) CFU-C inhibitors in aplastic anaemia. *Blut* **48(2):** 61–74.

Mortimer PP, Humphries RK, Moore JG, Purcell RH & Young NS (1983) A human parvovirus-like virus inhibits haematopoietic colony formation in vitro. *Nature* **302(5907):** 426–429.

Nago T & Maurer AM (1969) Concordance for drug induced aplastic anemia in identical twins. *New England Journal of Medicine* **281:** 11.

Nissen C, Iscove NN & Speck B (1979) High burst promoting activity (BPA) in serum of patients with acquired aplastic anemia. *Experimental Hematology Today* 1: 79–87.

Nissen C, Cornu P, Gratwohl A & Speck B (1980) Peripheral blood cells from patients with aplastic anaemia in partial remission suppress growth of their own bone marrow precursors in culture. *British Journal of Haematology* 45: 233–243.

Nissen C, Moser Y, Bürgin M et al (1982) Aplastic anemia: low production of hemopoietic growth factors predicts failure or retarded recovery after immunosuppressive treatment. *Experimental Hematology* 10 (supplement 12): 143–149.

Nissen C, Moser Y, Speck B & Bendy J (1983) Haemopoietic stimulators and inhibitors in aplastic anaemia serum. *British Journal of Haematology* 54: 519–530.

Nissen C, Moser Y, Speck B & Bendy J (1984) Soluble factors in aplastic anemia with hemolymphopoietic activity. In Young NS, Levine AS & Humphries RK (eds) *Aplastic Anemia. Stem Cell Biology and Advances in Treatment*, pp 107–118. New York: Alan Liss.

Nissen C, Moser Y, Weis J & Speck B (1985a) Stimulatory serum factors in aplastic anemia. Part I: Serum 'releaser' activity for hemopoietic growth factors, a regulator? *British Jounal of Haematology* 61: 491–498.

Nissen C, Moser Y, Speck B, Gratwohl A, Weis J (1985b) Stimulatory serum factors in aplastic anemia. Part II: Prognostic significance for patients treated with high dose immunosuppression. *British Journal of Haematology* 61: 499–512.

Nissen C, Moser Y, Weis J et al (1986a) The release of interleukin-2 (IL-2) and colony stimulating activity (CSA) in aplastic anemia patients: opposite behaviour with improvement of marrow function. *Blut* 52: 221–230.

Nissen C, Gratwohl A, Speck B et al (1986b) Acquired aplastic anaemia: a PNH-like disease? *British Journal of Haematology* 64: 355–362.

Odum N, Platz P, Morling N et al (1987) Increased frequency of HLA DPw3 in severe aplastic anaemia (AA). *Bone Marrow Transplantation* 2 (supplement 1): 116.

Ruiz-Arguelles GJ, Katzmann JA, Greipp PR et al (1984) Lymphocyte subsets in patients with aplastic anemia. *American Journal of Hematology* 16(3): 267–275.

Ruvidic R, Jovcic G, Biljanovic-Paunovic L et al (1985) Myelopoiesis and erythropoiesis of bone marrow cells cultured in vitro in patients recovered from aplastic anaemia. *Scandinavian Journal of Haematology* 35(4): 437–444.

Saarinen UM, Chorba TL, Tattersall P et al (1976) Human parvovirus B19 induced epidemic acute red cell aplasia in patients with hereditary hemolytic anemia *Blood* 67(5): 1411–1417.

Schultz DR, Walling JS & Yunis AA (1979) Evidence for an immune mechanism in chloramphenicol induced aplastic anemia. *Clinical Research* 27: 464A.

Singer JW, Brown JE, James MC et al (1978) Effect of peripheral blood lymphocytes from patients with aplastic anemia on granulocytic colony growth from HLA-matched and mismatched marrows: effect of transfusion sensitization. *Blood* 52: 37–46.

Suda T, Mizoguchi H, Miura Y, et al (1980) Enhancement of granulocytic colony formation by deletion of phagocytic cells in the bone marrow of patients with idiopathic aplastic anemia. *Experimental Hematology* 8(6): 659–665.

Suda T, Mizoguchi H, Miura Y, Kubota K & Takaku F (1981) Suppression of in vitro granulocyte-macrophage colony formation by the peripheral mononuclear phagocytic cells of patients with idiopathic aplastic anaemia. *British Journal of Haematology* 47: 433–442.

Sullivan R, Quesenberry PJ, Parkman R et al (1980) Aplastic anemia: lack of inhibitory effect of bone marrow lymphocytes on in vitro granulopoiesis. *Blood* 56(4): 625–632.

Takaku F, Suda T, Mizoguchi H et al (1980) Effect of peripheral blood mononuclear cells from aplastic anemia patients on the granulocyte-macrophage and erythroid colony formation in samples from normal human bone marrow in vitro—a cooperative work. *Blood* 55: 937–943.

Tichelli A, Gratwohl A, Würsch A, Nissen C & Speck B (1988) Leukaemia occurring after severe aplastic anaemia. *British Journal of Haematology* (in press).

Torok-Storb B (1984) T-cell effects on in vitro erythropoiesis: immune regulation and immune reactivity. *Progress in Clinical and Biology Research* 148: 163–172.

Torok-Storb BJ, Storb R, Graham TC et al (1978) Erythropoiesis in vitro: effect of normal versus 'transfusion-sensitized' mononuclear cells. *Blood* 52: 706–711.

Torok-Storb B, Sieff C, Storb R et al (1980) In vitro tests for distinguishing possible immune mediated aplastic anemia from transfusion induced sensitization. *Blood* 55(2): 211–215.

Torok-Storb B, Johnson GG, Bowden R & Storb R (1987) Gamma-interferon in aplastic anemia: inability to detect significant levels in sera or demonstrate hematopoietic suppressing activity. *Blood* **69(2):** 629–633.

Torres A, Gomez P, Alonso MC et al (1983) Lack of in vitro colony formation in a patient with severe aplastic anemia after spontaneous autologous hematologic reconstitution. *Acta Haematologica (Basel)* **70(1):** 63–67.

Wang WC, Herrod HG & Presbury GJ (1986) Lymphocyte subsets in children with aplastic anemia. *American Journal of Medical Sciences* **291(5):** 304–309.

Warren RR, Storb R, Thomas ED et al (1980) Autoimmune and alloimmune phenomena in patients with aplastic anemia: cytotoxicity against autologous lymphocytes and lymphocytes from HLA identical siblings. *Blood* **56:** 683–689.

Wiktor-Jedrzeijczak W, Siekierzynski M, Szczylik C, Gornas P & Dryjanski T (1982) Aplastic anemia with marrow defective in formation of fibroblastoid cell colonies in vitro. *Scandinavian Journal of Haematology* **28:** 82–90.

Wintrobe MM (1981) *Clinical Hematology*, 8th edn. Philadelphia: Lea & Febiger.

Yoshida K, Miura I, Takahashi T et al (1983) Quantitative and qualitative analysis of stem cells of patients with aplastic anemia. *Scandinavian Journal of Haematology* **30(4):** 317–323.

Young NS, Mortimer PP, Moore JG & Humphries RK (1984) Characterization of a virus that causes transient aplastic crisis. *Journal of Clinical Investigation* **73(1):** 224–230.

Yunis AA (1973) Chloramphenicol induced bone marrow suppression. *Seminars in Hematology* **10:** 225–234.

Yunis AA, Miller AM, Salem Z & Arimura GK (1980) Chloramphenicol toxicity: pathogenetic mechanisms and the role of p No2 in aplastic anemia. *Clinical Toxicology* **17(3):** 359–373.

Zoumbos NC, Ferris WO, Hsu SM et al (1984) Analysis of lymphocyte subsets in patients with aplastic anaemia. *British Journal of Haematology* **58(1):** 95–105.

Zoumbos NC, Gascon P, Djeu JY, Trost SR & Young NS (1985a) Circulating activated suppressor T-lymphocytes in aplastic anemia. *New England Journal of Medicine* **312:** 257–265.

Zoumbos NC, Gascon P, Djen JY & Young NS (1985b) Interferon is a mediator of hematopoietic suppression in aplastic anemia in vitro and possibly in vivo. *Proceedings of the National Academy of Sciences USA* **82:** 188–192.

4

Viruses and bone marrow failure

GARY KURTZMAN
NEAL YOUNG

That virus infection may cause serious bone marrow failure, long suspected by clinical association, has been confirmed by the recent demonstration of the interaction of specific viruses and haematopoietic cells. These laboratory advances, which have direct clinical importance, have been made possible by the application of molecular techniques for virus detection and by practical cell culture systems for the bone marrow. This article will review the relationship of several viruses to bone marrow failure: the viruses have been selected either because the mechanism of interaction is relatively well understood (Epstein–Barr virus, B19 parvovirus), or because the virus has been implicated as an agent of haematological disease in large populations (hepatitis, human immunodeficiency virus). Viruses and bone marrow failure is a topic that has been periodically reviewed (Camitta, 1979; Aymard et al, 1980; Young and Mortimer, 1984). The reader is particularly referred to a recent discussion on the complementary subject of the haematological consequences of common viral infections (Baranski and Young, 1987).

VIRUSES AND APLASTIC ANAEMIA

Clinical associations and epidemiology

Confident assignment of an aetiological agent to an individual case of aplastic anaemia is usually impossible; most cases are designated as 'idio-pathic'. Nonetheless, occasional patients with aplastic anaemia will have an obvious antecedent viral illness by history: infectious mononucleosis, hepatitis, or, in children, a severe febrile prodromal illness. Patients with hepatitis-associated disease are younger and more often male than for aplastic anaemia in general; these characteristics parallel those of populations of patients with viral hepatitis rather than primary bone marrow failure (Ajlouni and Doeblin, 1974; Camitta et al, 1974; Hagler et al, 1975). The peculiar global epidemiology of aplastic anaemia, with an apparently higher prevalence in the Orient compared to the West, also follows the distribution of hepatitis virus and other viruses and there may also be more cases of hepatitis-associated aplasia in the Far East (Young et al, 1986). The association of viral illness and aplasia may be underestimated because of the lack of a serological assay for non-A non-B hepatitis; perhaps as many as half of the patients presenting with aplastic anaemia have elevated serum transaminase levels.

Immune phenomena in aplastic anaemia

Because many patients with aplastic anaemia have responded haematologically to therapy directed at the immune system, such as antithymocyte and antilymphocyte globulins, the role of lymphocytes in haematopoietic failure has been intensively investigated. While the pathogenetic importance of immunological abnormalities in this disease is controversial, the immune cell dysfunction seen in aplastic anaemia patients is similar to that observed in man and in animals infected with viruses (Young, 1987; Baranski and Young, 1988). Patients with aplastic anaemia commonly have activated lymphocytes (both atypical lymphocytes on peripheral blood smear and cells bearing antigens like HLA-DR and the interleukin-2 receptor detected by flow cytometry study), inverted helper: suppressor lymphocyte ratios (due to a combination of decreased helper and increased suppressor cells), elevated serum levels of the soluble form of the interleukin-2 receptor, and increased and dysregulated production of the lymphokines interleukin-2 and γ-interferon.

Virus-associated haemophagocytic syndrome

This syndrome often presents with pancytopenia. The pathology of the bone marrow is characterized by the conspicuous phagocytosis of red cells, platelets, and nucleated cells by benign-appearing histiocytes (Risdall et al, 1979). (Erythrophagocytosis may also be present in aplastic bone marrows when sought.) The majority of patients have been previously immunosuppressed, historically by chemotherapy (renal transplant, maintenance treatment of malignant disease) and more recently in the acquired immunodeficiency syndrome (AIDS) (Spivak et al, 1984). The haemophagocytic syndrome has been observed during the course of infection with a number of different viruses, including cytomegalovirus Epstein–Barr virus, (EBV), herpes simplex, varicella-zoster, adenovirus and parainfluenza 1 (Risdall et al, 1979; Wilson et al, 1981; Yin et al, 1983; Morris et al, 1985; Sullivan et al, 1985; Tomomasa et al, 1986; Christensson et al, 1987). EBV has been directly demonstrated in the bone marrow of a few patients (Sullivan et al, 1985).

EPSTEIN–BARR VIRUS

Haematological abnormalities, particularly mild neutropenia, thrombocytopenia and haemolytic anaemia, during the course of infectious mononucleosis are common (Carter, 1965, 1966; Tronel et al, 1966). Severe aplastic anaemia following closely on infectious mononucleosis is clearly much rarer: only about a dozen patients have been reported in the literature (Lazarus and Baehner, 1981; Sullivan, 1984; Ahronheim et al, 1983; Sawaka et al, 1987). In the reported cases the diagnosis of infectious mononucleosis had been suggested by obvious symptoms and the presence of atypical lymphocytes and was confirmed serologically. Bone marrow failure usually occurred within a month of the onset of symptoms of EBV infection. Some patients have died as a result of the complications of pancytopenia, and others have recovered coincident with a variety of therapies (cortico-steroids, androgens, antithymocyte globulin).

Bone marrow failure in the setting of EBV infection probably occurs more frequently in abnormal clinical settings. In the peculiar X-linked lympho-proliferative syndrome, characterized by serology showing active EBV infection, hypogammaglobulinaemia and lymphocyte proliferation, some-times progressing to lymphoma, a large proportion (17/75 in one study) of affected boys apparently died of aplastic anaemia, although marrow cellu-larity has not been described in detail for most cases (Purtilo et al, 1982). A kindred study has also been described in which a high incidence of naso-pharyngeal carcinoma and aplastic anaemia has been credited to EBV infection (Schimke et al, 1987). Pancytopenia can also occur in other patients with sporadic chronic EBV infection, although the bone marrow morphology may show lymphocytic or histiocytic (see above) infiltration rather than acellularity. More limited lineage failure in the form of pure red cell aplasia has also been associated with EBV infection (Socinski et al, 1984).

Using molecular and immunological methods, we have identified EBV in the bone marrow of four patients with aplastic anaemia and two with pure red cell aplasia (Baranski et al, 1988). The index case was typical in that severe aplastic anaemia followed immediately on infectious mononucleosis; EBV was demonstrated in the residual bone marrow cells by immuno-fluorescence for Epstein–Barr nuclear antigen (EBNA) and by in situ hybridization and Southern blot analysis using EBV-specific probes. EBV was not present in peripheral blood cells or in the bone marrow of normal and haematological controls, including one patient with uncomplicated acute infectious mononucleosis. EBV infection manifested as infectious mononucleosis was also associated with pure red cell aplasia in two patients with probably limited red cell reserves—one patient with Diamond–Blackfan syndrome in remission and another with sickle cell anaemia (Baranski, unpublished observations). In two patients with aplastic anaemia, preceding EBV infection was not clinically obvious. One patient was identified retrospectively in a survey of 30 stored DNA samples from patients with aplastic anaemia.

Mechanisms of EBV-associated marrow failure

EBV infection of B lymphocytes leads to their polyclonal activation, with hypergammaglobulinaemia and increased circulating immunoglobulin-secreting cells. In response there is proliferation of activated T lymphocytes, especially of the suppressor phenotype, CD 8, associated with increased circulating soluble interleukin-2 receptor, and increased interferon production (Tosato et al, 1979; Tomkinson et al, 1987; Tosato, 1987). Similar immunological abnormalities have been described in aplastic anaemia, and the suppressor cell may have a pathogenetic role in bone marrow inhibition (see above). Cells expressing the CD 8 antigen (lymphocytes or natural killer cells) have also been implicated in neutropenia, anaemia and thrombocytopenia associated with chronic T-γ lymphoproliferative disorders (Reynolds and Foon, 1984). Occasional patients with EBV-associated aplastic anaemia appear to have responded to antithymocyte globulin (Swaka et al, 1987; Baranski et al, 1988).

In some cases mononuclear cells from the blood of infectious mononucleosis patients or from the bone marrow of EBV-induced marrow failure patients have suppressed normal haematopoiesis in vitro (Shadduck et al, 1979; Gardner et al, 1986). In a patient with EBV-associated pure red cell aplasia, T-cell depletion restored in vitro erythropoiesis (Socinski et al, 1984). We have generated activated T lymphocytes by exposure to EBV or to autologous EBV-infected B lymphocytes; these activated T-cells can inhibit autologous haematopoiesis in colony culture (Baranski et al, unpublished observations). These activated T-cells produce interferon and thus may inhibit cell proliferation non-specifically; in addition, they inhibit haematopoiesis from EBV-exposed autologous bone marrow cells more efficiently than uninfected cells.

While B cells are the recognized target of EBV infection, other cells may also harbour this virus (for example, nasopharyngeal epithelial cells). Some haematopoietic cells may also be infected by EBV, since EBNA by immunofluorescence and EBV DNA sequences by hybridization have been detected in B-cell-depleted normal bone marrow after exposure to purified virus (Baranski et al, unpublished observations). The usual strains of EBV are not inhibitory of normal haematopoiesis in vitro, but EBV-exposed cells may be more susceptible to T-cell-mediated cytotoxicity. However, EBV isolated from patients with aplastic anaemia has had molecular and biological properties associated with a cytolytic, non-transforming strain, in contrast to the usual transforming EBV commonly obtained from infected persons (Baranski et al, 1988).

Why EBV only rarely results in marrow failure remains unclear. Possible explanations include a defective virus more toxic than the normal type that directly infects the haematopoietic stem cell; an unusual suppressive lymphocyte response genetically or randomly determined in the host's immune response; or a predisposing defect in the haematopoietic stem cell compartment making it more susceptible to either virus or immune response.

B19 PARVOVIRUS

Parvoviruses are common agents of animal disease. The B19 parvovirus was discovered in 1975 in the sera of normal blood bank donors (Cossart et al, 1975); seroepidemiological studies have linked acute infection with this

5

Bone marrow aplasia due to radiation accidents: pathophysiology, assessment and treatment

RICHARD CHAMPLIN

Radionuclides are increasingly utilized in medicine, science and industry. Nuclear energy is extensively used to produce electricity and for weapons. Accidental or unintentional exposure to radiation has become a frequent problem. The recent accidents at the nuclear power station in Chernobyl (USSR State Committee on the Utilization of Atomic Energy, 1986; US Nuclear Regulatory Commission, 1987) and related to an abandoned medical radiation therapy source in Goiania, Brazil (Roberts, 1987) emphasize the need for the medical community to understand the pathophysiology, assessment and treatment of radiation injuries. This review will primarily focus on the effects of whole body radiation exposure.

The sensitivity to cytotoxicity from radiation varies among cell types and tissues (Hubner and Fry, 1980; United Nations, 1982, 1985; Bond and Cronkite, 1986). The dose-response effects have been reviewed (United Nations, 1985). The bone marrow is the most sensitive critical tissue to the effects of radiation. With increasing doses, the gastrointestinal tract, skin, lungs and other tissues are also affected. In general, radiation is most toxic to rapidly proliferating cells and cells that must undergo multiple divisions (Bond et al, 1965; United Nations, 1985). Progenitor and precursor cells such as haematopoietic stem cells of the bone marrow, mucosal crypt cells of gastrointestinal tract and basal epithelial cells of the skin are more sensitive than the mature non-proliferating cells of these tissues. The fully mature cells of these organs are not lysed by radiation doses typically experienced with accidental exposures; therefore, the effects of radiation injury are not fully manifest until after these cells pass through their normal life span. Maximum organ damage becomes evident as the injured progenitor cells fail to replace the lost mature cells. Lymphocytes are an exception to this rule; they are rapidly lysed by radiation and undergo interphase death. Whole body radiation rapidly produces profound lymphocytopenia and immunosuppression (Wald, 1983; Barabanova et al, 1984; United Nations, 1985; Bond and Cronkite, 1986).

The dose-response effects of accidental whole body radiation exposure are poorly defined in man due to the small number of documented cases in which an accurate determination of the absorbed dose could be made. Radiation injury is dependent on a number of factors, including the type and quality of radiation, dose, dose rate, homogeneity of the dose and shielding. Higher doses can be tolerated if given over a protracted period (Mole, 1984a). The World Health Organization and other groups have accumulated data on several hundred victims of radiation exposure, allowing several tentative conclusions to be drawn (Rubin and Casarett, 1968; Barabanova et al, 1984; United Nations, 1985).

Doses of radiation exceeding 1.5–2 Gy produce bone marrow hypoplasia by cytotoxicity to haematopoietic stem cells (Bond et al, 1965; Wald, 1971, 1983; United Nations, 1985; Bond and Cronkite, 1986). This leads to pancytopenia and immunosuppression, predisposing victims to opportunistic infections and bleeding which typically occur 2–4 weeks after the exposure. Increasing doses of radiation produce a lower nadir in circulating granulocytes, erythrocytes and platelets and a longer duration of pancytopenia. The bone marrow microenvironment is not damaged in doses experienced in most radiation accidents. With very high doses of radiation, exceeding 30 Gy, the microenvironment is affected and can no longer support haematopoiesis.

The $LD_{50/60}$, the lethal dose to 50% of exposed individuals within 60 days, is a commonly used measure of mortality due to bone marrow suppression. Following the Hiroshima atomic bomb explosion when only limited medical care was available, the $LD_{50/60}$ due to radiation was estimated to be 2.2–3.0 Gy (United Nations, 1985; Solomon and Marston, 1986). If optimal supportive medical care is administered, including antibiotics and blood product transfusions, the LD_{50} for total body irradiation is approximately 4.5 Gy and there is approximately 90% mortality at doses of 7 Gy (United Nations, 1985; Gale, 1987). With higher doses, generally exceeding 10–12 Gy, severe toxicity to the gastrointestinal tract and other organs ensues (Wilson, 1959; Keane et al, 1981). Injury to the gastrointestinal epithelium by high doses of radiation leads to denudation of the mucosa, massive diarrhoea and sepsis, typically resulting in death within 6–9 days of exposure. Very high doses of total body irradiation exceeding 50 Gy produce neurotoxicity and cardiovascular collapse which is fatal within several days

Table 1. Medical considerations for accidental whole body radiation.

Assessment
  Nature of accident, types of radiation
  Extent of exposure
  Associated injuries

Limitation of exposure
  Evacuation
  Debridement/decontamination

Dose estimation

Supportive care and treatment
  Bone marrow failure
  Skin injuries
  Visceral injuries

Evaluation for late complications

(Fanger and Lushbaugh, 1967). Several major considerations must be made for the evaluation and treatment for victims of accidental radiation exposure (Table 1).

ASSESSMENT

The initial concern is to assess the nature of the accident, including the type of radiation and the extent of exposure. The most common radiation injuries are localized exposures to external radiation, most often to the hands or extremities of nuclear and medical radiation workers (Jamnet et al, 1986). This may produce serious injury to the irradiated region, but will not affect other shielded tissues.

In nuclear power station accidents such as the Chernobyl disaster there can be a tremendous release of radioactive materials into the environment. Victims are exposed to external and internal sources of whole body radiation. External radiation consists of beta, gamma and sometimes neutron radiation emitted from the plume of released radionuclides. Beta radiation is low-energy electrons which penetrate only 1–2 cm but can produce severe skin injuries. Gamma radiation is high-energy X-rays which penetrate through the body and can produce visceral complications. Neutron radiation exposure may also occur, although this was not an important factor in the Chernobyl accident (USSR State Committee on the Utilization of Atomic Energy, 1986). Internal radiation occurs from absorption of inhaled or ingested radionuclides, resulting in prolonged radiation exposure to the involved tissues (Voelz, 1980).

At Chernobyl, the most seriously affected victims were the power plant workers on duty at the time of the accident and firemen called in to control multiple fires that occurred after the explosion. They were primarily affected by external radiation with only a minor component of internal radiation exposure. Individuals on the scene were also subject to skin contamination from air-borne radioactive debris. There were also severe associated injuries that are not directly related to radiation, such as trauma from an explosion or thermal burns from associated fires. These associated injuries, particularly burns, substantially increase the mortality of radiation injuries (Brooks et al, 1952). The population in the region surrounding the Chernobyl reactor did not receive high enough doses to develop acute radiation sickness but a 30 km radius was evacuated because of concern for long-term effects (USSR State Committee on the Utilization of Atomic Energy, 1986, US Nuclear Regulatory Commission, 1987).

The recent accident in Goiania, Brazil, was an example involving external and high-dose internal radiation exposure (Roberts, 1987). This accident resulted from breakage of the casing of an abandoned radiation therapy source spilling 1400 Ci of caesium[137] in a junkyard. Children and adults were fascinated by the luminescent powder, including a number who rubbed it on their bodies or ate it; 244 people were reported to be contaminated. Substantial internal contamination in many victims exposed them to protracted whole body radiation. Treatment with chelating agents was unsuccessful, and at least four people died from marrow aplasia and infection.

In dealing with nuclear or radiation accidents in which large numbers of people have been exposed, it is critical to determine which victims have received sufficient doses of whole body exposure to require hospitalization for treatment of acute radiation sickness and bone marrow failure. Several proposals for evaluation and triage have been reported (Andrews, 1980; Ricks, 1980; Doege et al, 1986; Saenger, 1986).

The primary factors to consider are gastrointestinal symptoms, cutaneous effects and depression of peripheral blood counts. Doses of whole body radiation less than 50–100 rem generally do not produce acute symptoms. Higher doses produce acute radiation sickness. The most prominent symptoms are anorexia, nausea and vomiting. The interval from exposure to symptoms is inversely related to the radiation dose, although there is considerable variability. Victims complaining of nausea within 24 hours of radiation exposure require careful evaluation. A baseline complete blood count should be promptly obtained in all exposed individuals and repeated daily for 3 days. Those with protracted gastrointestinal symptoms, cutaneous erythema or lymphocyte counts $<1.5 \times 10^9/l$ within the first 2–3 days require hospitalization. Others should be followed with weekly examinations, including complete blood counts for at least 1 month.

Dose-dependent haematological effects

In many radiation accidents, exposed individuals are not wearing a monitoring device capable of accurately measuring high doses of external radiation. It is necessary to estimate the radiation dose in these cases based upon its biological effects. Haematological parameters can be utilized for biological dosimetry assuming uniform whole body irradiation (Wald, 1983;

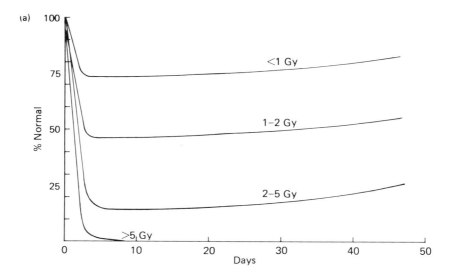

Barabanova et al, 1984; Eisert and Mendelsohn, 1984). Dose-dependent changes in haematopoietic cells are shown in Figure 1. The earliest indicator is the lymphocyte count. Whole body radiation rapidly produces lymphocytopenia. The rate of fall in circulating lymphocytes is directly related to the whole body radiation dose (Cronkite, 1951) and is a relatively accurate guide for doses up to 3 Gy. With higher doses, profound lymphocytopenia

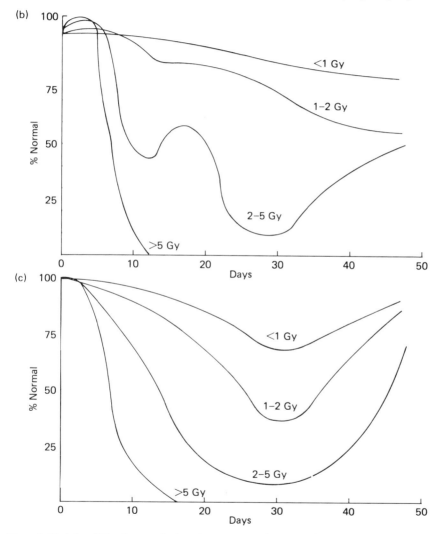

Figure 1. Peripheral blood counts for lymphocytes, granulocytes and platelets following various doses of whole body radiation. Data adapted from Wald (1971) and United Nations (1985). Victims receiving doses >5 Gy generally die of infection due to granulocytopenia or thrombocytopenic haemorrhage, although some will recover with optimal supportive care. (a) Lymphocytes; (b) granulocytes; (c) platelets.

occurs and the lymphocyte count is less reliable for estimating the radiation dose (Bond and Cronkite, 1986). Peripheral granulocytes are then a more accurate blood parameter for dose estimation. Unlike lymphocytes, granulocytes are not directly lysed by radiation. There is a large storage pool of granulocytes in the bone marrow; these cells must be mobilized and consumed before granulocytopenia will ensue. In individuals receiving 2–5 Gy, there is typically an abortive rise in the peripheral granulocyte count at approximately day 10, followed by a progressive fall to the true nadir. The nadir in the granulocyte count will typically occur between 8 to 30 days following radiation exposure (Wald, 1971; Barabanova et al, 1984). Higher doses result in increasingly severe granulocytopenia and a shorter interval from exposure to the nadir. Dose estimates based upon granulocytes are less affected by associated injuries and complications than are estimates by lymphocyte count. The severity of thrombocytopenia and reticulocytopenia are also indicators of radiation dose (Chaudhuri and Messerschmidt, 1982; Eisert and Mendelsohn, 1984).

Cytogenetics can also be used to estimate the dose of whole body radiation (Eisert and Mendelsohn, 1984; International Atomic Energy Agency, 1986). Radiation induces several characteristic chromosome abnormalities, particularly dicentric chromosomes. By scoring the frequency of these abnormalities in blood or bone marrow, a relatively accurate dose estimation can be made. An index of several factors can be used, improving dose estimation (Barabanova et al, 1984).

Other measurements have also been proposed to estimate whole body radiation dose, including total body ^{24}Na content (Mole, 1984b), electron spin resonance spectroscopy (Sagstuen et al, 1983) and somatic mutations involving glycophorin A (Hakoda et al, 1986) and hypoxanthine guanine phosphoribosyltransferase (Langlois et al, 1987).

SUPPORTIVE CARE AND EMERGENCY TREATMENT

Limitation of exposure

The initial therapeutic measure is to prevent further radiation exposure by promptly evacuating victims from the source of radiation. If possible, patients should be rushed to an emergency facility specifically designed to deal with contaminated radiation accident victims (Andrews, 1980; Ricks, 1980; Schlein, 1983; Saenger, 1986). Contaminated clothing should be removed and the skin rigorously bathed and decontaminated. Skin wounds should be meticulously debrided of any radioactive materials. If radionuclides have been ingested, emetic agents and purgatives should usually be employed. Chelating agents may be useful for some radionuclides (Voelz, 1980; Schlein, 1983). Pulmonary lavage has been proposed after inhalation of plutonium. ^{131}I is usually the most plentiful radionuclide produced by nuclear weapons and nuclear reactor accidents. The uptake of this nuclide by the thyroid can be blocked by administering large doses of non-radioactive iodine. This may reduce the potential risks of hypothyroidism and thyroid cancer (Becker, 1987).

Supportive treatment

Radioactive victims who develop pancytopenia require supportive care similar to that utilized for patients with aplastic anaemia or bone marrow failure from other aetiologies. Treatment measures are summarized in Table 2. Infections and bleeding are major causes of morbidity and mortality

Table 2. Management of bone marrow failure due to radiation accidents.

Protective isolation
  Low bacterial diet
  Prophylactic antibiotics
  Laminar airflow environment or reverse isolation

Treatment of infection
  Antibiotics—Gram-negative and -positive bacteria
  Antifungals—*Candida*, aspergillosis
  Antivirals—herpes simplex, cytomegalovirus

Blood products
  Red blood cell transfusions
  Platelet transfusions

Treatment to restore haematopoiesis
  Bone marrow transplantation
  Haematopoietic growth factors

(Bodey et al, 1966). Measures to limit acquisition of pathogenic bacteria include protective isolation and prophylactic oral antibiotics (Winston et al, 1986). Use of a laminar airflow environment may delay development of infection but its efficacy in improving survival has not been established (Buckner et al, 1978). Granulocytopenic patients developing fever require prompt treatment with empirical antibiotics designed to cover enteric bacteria, such as a semisynthetic penicillin (e.g. piperacillin) in combination with either an aminoglycoside or third-generation cephalosporin (Winston et al, 1986). Recrudescence of oral herpes simplex infection is common following whole body radiation and can be prevented or treated with acyclovir (Saral et al, 1981). Fungal infections frequently occur in patients with protracted granulocytopenia; diagnosis of these infections may be difficult and empirical treatment with amphotericin B is generally warranted for patients with fever unresponsive to broad-spectrum antibacterial antibiotics or who initially respond but develop recurrent fever (Winston et al, 1986).

Spontaneous bleeding may occur in patients with severe thrombocytopenia, and platelet transfusions are indicated to maintain a platelet count greater than $20 \times 10^9/l$. Erythrocyte transfusions should be administered to prevent symptoms of anaemia; it is advisable to maintain the haematocrit level $\geqslant 30\%$ to provide a margin of safety if major haemorrhage develops.

Care of skin injuries requires debridement, decontamination and topical care similar to that necessary for severe thermal burns. Skin grafts may be required (Stern, 1980; Jamnet et al, 1986). The gastrointestinal syndrome is extremely difficult to manage. Diarrhoea and fluid depletion must be managed with intravenous fluids and electrolyte replacement (Andrews, 1980). Since oral intake is typically impaired by mucositis and gastrointestinal intolerance, intravenous hyperalimentation is usually required. Unfortunately, because of damage to the bowel mucosa, severe bleeding and sepsis shock from enteric organisms generally ensue and few severely affected patients survive.

The results of the Chernobyl disaster illustrate that most victims receiving less than 4 Gy whole body irradiation will recover if treated with optimal supportive care. Mortality increases dramatically with higher doses of radiation and few patients receiving greater than 6 Gy survive (USSR State Committee on the Utilization of Atomic Energy, 1986).

TREATMENT TO RESTORE HAEMATOPOIESIS

Bone marrow transplantation

Despite optimal supportive care, most victims receiving >5–6 Gy of whole body radiation will not survive long enough to have haematological recovery. Bone marrow transplantation can rescue experimental animals from lethal whole body radiation (Broerse et al, 1978; Solomon and Marston, 1986; Monroy et al, in press). Based on these data high dose total body radiation and bone marrow transplantation have been used to treat aplastic anaemia, leukaemias and other cancers. Human leukaemia patients routinely receive treatment with 10–15.75 Gy of total body irradiation and recover with donor-derived haematopoiesis following bone marrow transplantation. Total body irradiation produces immunosuppression as well as myelosuppression and a sufficiently high dose of irradiation will prevent bone marrow graft rejection and allow stable engraftment. The minimum dose of whole body irradiation necessary to allow engraftment of human bone marrow transplants is poorly defined but exceeds 5 Gy; it depends on several factors, including the immunological competence of the recipient, the genetic disparity between donor and recipient and the source, nature and number of transplanted haematopoietic cells (Thomas et al, 1970; Vriesendorp, 1985). In animals, supralethal radiation is required. The dose of irradiation necessary to allow sustained engraftment is higher than the lethal whole body radiation (Broerse et al, 1978; Solomon and Marston, the donor and recipient are mismatched for major histocompatibility antigens and more intensive immunosuppressive treatment is necessary to achieve engraftment (Storb et al, 1983).

Bone marrow transplantation may be associated with a number of serious complications (Champlin and Gale, 1984). Graft rejection may occur if the recipient's immunity is not sufficiently suppressed. Immunocompetent lymphocytes present in the donor's bone marrow may react against recipient (host) tissues and produce graft versus host disease. Severe immunodeficiency inevitably occurs for 6–12 months following bone marrow transplantation before immunity is restored by cells derived from the donor bone marrow. Immunosuppressive treatments used to prevent or treat graft versus host disease may produce toxicity and further predispose patients to infection. A variety of opportunistic infections may occur following bone marrow transplantation. The most frequent fatal infection is interstitial pneumonitis caused by cytomegalovirus. A total of 20–30% of patients receiving bone marrow transplants from human leukocyte antigen (HLA)-identical donors as treatment for haematological diseases will die from one or more of these transplant-related complications; the risk increases substantially with transplants from HLA-non-identical donors (Beatty et al, 1985).

Bone marrow transplantation is a logical treatment for carefully selected victims of accidental total body irradiation who receive a sufficiently high dose that they are unlikely to have spontaneous marrow recovery. Bone marrow transplantation has a number of limitations, however, and is likely to benefit only a minority of patients (Champlin, 1987; Table 3). Identifi-

Table 3. Limitations on the use of bone marrow transplantation for nuclear accidents.

1. Applicable only to a small fraction of victims receiving high doses of radiation likely to produce lethal bone marrow failure but not lethal injury to other tissues
2. Difficulties with histocompatibility testing due to lymphocytopenia
3. Lack of an HLA-identical related donor for most patients
4. Requirements for additional immunosuppressive therapy
5. Results related to age; few survivors > 50 years of age
6. Risk of transplant-related complications, rejection, graft versus host disease, post-transplant immunodeficiency
7. Complications of radiation injury to other tissues

cation of a histocompatible donor is difficult. High dose total body irradiation rapidly produces lymphocytopenia making HLA-typing difficult; serological typing to the HLA-A, B, and C loci can generally be accomplished, but insufficient numbers of lymphocytes are usually present to allow mixed lymphocyte culture and HLA D region typing. The best results have been achieved with transplants from an HLA-identical sibling donor, but a matched sibling is available for only one third of victims. Ideally, unrelated HLA-identical donors could be utilized, but there are several major logistical problems. Complete HLA-typing is required. Due to the tremendous polymorphism of the HLA gene complex the probability of any two unrelated individuals being HLA-identical is small, and it is necessary to screen approximately 100 000 potential donors to have an 80% chance of identifying a histocompatible donor (US Office of Technology Assessment, 1987). Several large donor registries have recently been established, but these searches are often unsuccessful and are too time-consuming to be practical in an emergency setting, particularly given the problems in performed complete histocompatibility typing. The dose of accidental whole body radiation exposure, although life-threatening, may not provide sufficient immunosuppression to prevent graft rejection, particularly for HLA-non-identical transplants. Use of additional immunosuppressive treatment is necessary; this introduces the potential for drug toxicity and increases the risk of opportunistic infections.

Results with bone marrow transplants are age-related; the best results occur in children and young adults. Few patients greater than 50 years of age survive following bone marrow transplantation (Klingemann et al, 1986). At mid-lethal doses, histoincompatible bone marrow transplantation has been reported to be associated with increased mortality in mice, a phenomenon termed the mid-zone effect and related to graft rejection (Trentin, 1959). This mid-zone effect has not been documented in dogs (Monroy et al, in press) or in man. In other animal models, survival is improved by transplantation of haploidentical T-cell-depleted bone marrow even without sustained engraftment. Transient engraftment and haematological recovery may be protective until autologous marrow recovery can occur (Ferrera et al, 1987).

Victims of nuclear reactor accidents often suffer severe trauma and skin burns in addition to radiation exposure. Most victims of the Chernobyl accident who received a sufficiently high dose of irradiation to be considered for bone marrow transplantation had thermal burns as well as life-threatening radiation injuries to skin, gastrointestinal tract, lungs or other tissues. Because of the severe nature of these associated injuries, most of these victims were ineligible to receive transplants or died prior to the time necessary for bone marrow transplant to engraft and produce haematological recovery (USSR State Committee on the Utilization of Atomic Energy, 1986).

Thirteen victims of the Chernobyl nuclear accident who were exposed to radiation greater than 5 Gy received bone marrow transplants (USSR State Committee on the Utilization of Atomic Energy, 1986; Ferrera et al, 1987). An HLA-identical donor was only available for 7 patients, and 6 received haploidentical-related transplants. Of the 13 bone marrow transplant recipients, 7 died of skin burns, gastrointestinal toxicity and infections within 3 weeks. Six patients survived long enough to have haematological recovery, but 4 died of later infections. There is concern that graft versus host disease may have contributed to the death of 2 patients. Two transplant recipients survived; these patients had transient engraftment of donor cells followed by recovery of autologous haematopoiesis. No donor could be identified for another 9 of the most seriously affected patients; these patients received haematopoietic cells from an unrelated fetal liver but died shortly thereafter from radiation injury to the skin, gastrointestinal tract and other tissues (USSR State Committee on the Utilization of Atomic Energy, 1986).

The role of bone marrow transplantation in the treatment of nuclear disaster victims is controversial, and there is little previous experience to support firm recommendations. Mathe and co-workers (1959) performed marrow transplantation for four victims of a 1958 nuclear reactor accident in Yugoslavia; these transplants were performed approximately 1 month after exposure and none of the patients had sustained engraftment. Thomas et al reported one patient who recovered following transplantation of bone marrow from an identical twin; it is impossible to determine whether the patient had engraftment of the donor marrow or whether he recovered autologous haematopoiesis; the prompt recovery suggested a benefit from transplantation (Gilberti, 1980).

Bone marrow transplantation should be used when the anticipated benefit outweighs its risk. The precise indications for bone marrow transplantation as treatment for nuclear accidents are uncertain and one cannot simply extrapolate from the indications for aplastic anaemia or other haematological disorders. Some victims will slowly recover haematopoiesis, although pancytopenic patients cannot typically survive for a protracted period without haematological recovery. Many radiation accident victims also have severe radiation injury to non-haematopoietic tissues, particularly the skin and gastrointestinal tract; conceivably, occurrence of a superimposed transplant-related complication, such as graft versus host disease, could be lethal in these debilitated patients. Bone marrow transplantation should be more effective in accidents in which thermal burns and radiation-induced skin and visceral injuries are less prominent; situations more similar to the 'therapeutic' whole body radiation exposure used with bone marrow transplants for treatment of leukaemia. Most patients lack an HLA-identical related donor and the indications for unrelated HLA-identical or related HLA-non-identical transplants are even more difficult to determine since graft rejection or severe graft versus host disease are more likely with increasing genetic disparity.

Bone marrow transplantation can only benefit a small fraction of victims from radiation accidents—those who receive a total body radiation dose that is likely to produce death from bone marrow aplasia without life-threatening injury to other tissues. Given the experience with the Chernobyl victims, transplants should probably be considered for victims receiving more than 7–8 Gy but not in victims receiving lower doses. A number of important factors require clarification and further study in animals, including the optimal interval from exposure to transplantation and the requirement for additional immunosuppressive therapy, particularly for recipients of HLA-non-identical transplants. The efficacy of T-cell depletion to prevent graft versus host disease and the use of unrelated HLA-identical donors for bone marrow transplantation is under active evaluation in patients with other haematological diseases. If techniques can be developed to ensure engraftment without graft versus host disease, it would greatly improve the efficacy of bone marrow transplantation for radiation victims.

Haematopoietic growth factors

Doses of whole body radiation up to 12 Gy do not completely ablate haematopoiesis. Small numbers of lymphoid cells and haematopoietic progenitors persist (Buttarini et al, 1986), although patients receiving >6 Gy generally succumb to infections or bleeding before haematopoiesis can recover. Several haematopoietic growth factors have been cloned and produced for clinical trials (Metcalf, 1985). Granulocyte colony-stimulating factor (G-CSF) and granulocyte-macrophage colony-stimulating factor (GM-CSF) induce leukocytosis in animals and in man (Nienhuis et al, 1977; Donahue et al, 1986; Groopman et al, 1987). These agents increase the rate of haematopoietic recovery after chemotherapy and radiation and after bone marrow transplantation (Nienhuis et al, 1977). GM-CSF was used for treatment of severely affected victims in the Goiania accident, resulting in improvement in haematopoiesis (Buttarini et al, 1988). The gene for human interleukin-3, which stimulates myeloid, erythroid and megakaryocytic cells, has recently been cloned (Yang et al, 1986) and this growth factor will soon be entering clinical trials. Preliminary data in monkeys suggest that combination of interleukin-3 plus later acting factors such as GM-CSF will have synergistic effects (Donahue et al, 1987). It is likely that treatment with these agents will enhance the rate of haematopoietic recovery in radiation accident victims and may obviate the need for bone marrow transplantation in high dose radiation victims. Although promising, critical evaluation of these agents is necessary to determine whether survival will be improved for radiation victims with bone marrow failure.

REFERENCES

Andrews GA (1980) Management of accidental total body irradiation. In Hubner KF & Fry SA *The Medical Basis of Radiation Accident Preparedness*, pp 297–301. Amsterdam: Elsevier/North Holland.

Barabanova AV, Baronov AK, Guskova A et al (1984) Acute radiation effects in man. Submission of the Russian delegation to UNSCEAR.

Beatty PG, Clift RA, Michelson EM et al (1985) Marrow transplantation from related donors other HLA-identical siblings. *New England Journal of Medicine* **313:** 765–771.

Becker DV (1987) Reactor accidents: public health strategies and their medical implications. *Journal of the American Medical Association* **258:** 649–654.

Bodey GP, Buckley M, Sathe YS & Friereich EJ (1966) Quantitative relationship between circulating leukocytes and infections in patients with acute leukemia. *Annals of Internal Medicine* **64:** 328–340.

Bond VP & Cronkite EP (1986) *Workshop on Short-term Health Effects of Reactor Accidents: Chernobyl.* Report BNL 52030. US Dept of Energy.

Bond VP, Fliedner TM & Archambeau JO (1965) *Mammalian Radiation Lethality: a Disturbance in Cellular Kinetics.* New York: Academic Press.

Broerse JJ, von Bekkum DW, Hollander CF et al (1978) Mortality of monkeys after exposure to fission neutrons and the effects of autologous bone marrow transplantation. *International Journal of Radiation Biology* **34:** 253–264.

Brooks JW, Evans EI, Han WT & Reid JD (1952) The influence of external body radiation on mortality from thermal burns. *Annals of Surgery* **136:** 533–545.

Buckner CD, Clift RA, Sanders JE et al (1978) Protective environment for marrow transplant recipients. *Annals of Internal Medicine* 893–901.

Buttarini A, Seeger R & Gale RP (1986) Recipient immune competent T-lymphocytes can survive intensive conditioning for bone marrow transplantation. *Blood* **68:** 954–956.

Buttarini A, DeSouza PC, Gale RP et al (1988) Use of recombinant granulocyte-macrophage colony stimulating factor in the Brazil radiation accident. *Lancet* **2:** 471–475.

Champlin RE (1987) Role of bone marrow transplantation for nuclear accidents: implications of the Chernobyl disaster. *Seminars in Hematology* **24 (supplement 2):** 1–4.

Champlin RE & Gale RP (1984) Early complications of bone marrow transplantation. *Seminars in Hematology* **21:** 101–108.

Chaudhuri JP & Messerschmidt O (1982) Amount of peripheral reticulocytes as biologic dosimetry of ionizing radiation: experiments in the rabbit. *Acta Radiologica et Oncologica* **21:** 177–179.

Cronkite EP (1951) Hematology, diagnosis and therapy of radiation injury. *US Armed Forces Medical Journal* **56:** 661–669.

Doege TC, Wheater RH & Hendee WR (eds) (1986) *Proceedings of the International Confer-*

ence on Non-military Radiation Emergencies. Washington, DC: American Medical Association.

Donahue RE, Wang EA, Stone DK et al (1986) Stimulation of haematopoiesis in primates by continuous infusion of recombinant human GM-CSF. *Nature* **321:** 872–875.

Donahue RE, Seehra J, Norton C et al (1987) Stimulation of hematopoiesis in primates with human interleukin-3 and granulocyte, macrophage colony-stimulating factor. *Blood* **70 (supplement 1):** 133a.

Eisert WG & Mendelsohn ML (eds) (1984) *Biological Dosimetry.* Berlin: Springer-Verlag.

Fanger H & Lushbaugh CC (1967) Radiation death from cardiovascular shock following a criticality accident: report of a second death from a newly defined human radiation death syndrome. *Archives of Pathology and Laboratory Medicine* **83:** 446–460.

Ferrera J, Lipton J, Hellman S, Burakoff S & Mauck P (1987) Engraftment following T cell depleted marrow transplantation. *Transplantation* **43:** 461–467.

Gale RP (1987) Immediate medical consequences of nuclear accidents. *Journal of the American Medical Association* **258:** 625–628.

Gilberti MV (1987) The 1967 radiation accident near Pittsburg, Pennsylvania and a follow up report. In Hubner KF, Fry SA (eds) *Medical Basis for Radiation Accident Preparedness,* pp 131–140. Amsterdam: Elsevier (North Holland).

Groopman JE, Mitsuyasu RT, DeLeo MJ, Oette DH & Golde DW (1987) Effect of recombinant human granulocyte-macrophage colony-stimulating factor on myelopoiesis in the acquired immunodeficiency syndrome. *New England Journal of Medicine* **317:** 593–598.

Hakoda M, Akiyama M, Tatsugawa K et al (1986) Mutant 6-TG resistant T-lymphocytes in the peripheral blood of A-bomb survivors: I. Measurement of their frequency. *Journal of Radiation Research* **27:** 89.

Hubner KF & Fry SA (eds) (1980) *Medical Basis for Nuclear Accident Preparedness.* Amsterdam: Elsevier/North Holland.

International Atomic Energy Agency (1986) *Biological Dosimetry: Chromosomal Aberration Analysis for Dose Assessment.* Technical report 260. Vienna: International Atomic Energy Agency.

Jamnet H, Daburon F, Gerber GB, Hopewell JW, Haybittle JL & Whitfield L (eds) (1986) Radiation damage to the skin. *British Journal of Radiology* **(supplement 19)**.

Keane TJ, van Dyke J, Rider WD et al (1981) Idiopathic interstitial pneumonia following bone marrow transplantation: the relationship with total body irradiation. *International Journal of Radiation Oncology Biology Physics* **7:** 1365–1370.

Klingemann HG, Storb R & Fefer A (1986) Bone marrow transplantation in patients aged 45 years and older. *Blood* **67:** 770–776.

Langlois RG, Bigbee WL, Kyoizumi S et al (1987) Evidence for increased somatic cell mutations at the glycophorin A locus in atomic bomb survivors. *Science* **236:** 445–448.

Mathe G, Jammet H, Pendic B et al (1959) Transfusions et greffes de moelle osseuse homologue chez des humans irradiés à haute dose accidentellement. *Revue Française de l'Etude Clinique et Biologique* **4:** 226–238.

Metcalf D (1985) The granulocyte-macrophage colony-stimulating factors. *Science* **229:** 16–22.

Mole RH (1984a) Quantitative aspects of the lethal action of whole-body irradiation in the human species: brief and protracted exposure and the applicability of information from other mammalian species. *International Journal of Radiation Biology* **46:** 212–213.

Mole RH (1984b) Sodium in man and the assessment of radiation dose after criticality accidents. *Physical Medicine and Biology* **29:** 1307–1327.

Monroy RL, Vriesendorp HM & MacVittie TJ (1987) Improved survival of dogs exposed to fission neutron irradiation and transplanted with HLA identical bone marrow. *Bone Marrow Transplantation* **2:** 375–384.

Nienhuis AW, Donahue RE, Karlsson S et al (1977) Recombinant human granulocyte-macrophage colony stimulating factor (GM-CSF) shortens the period of neutropenia following autologous bone marrow transplantation in a primate model. *Journal of Clinical Investigation* **80:** 573–577.

Ricks RC (1980) REAC/TS: its role as a specialty referral center and training site. In Hubner KF & Fry SA (eds) *The Medical Basis of Radiation Accident Preparedness,* pp 291–296. Amsterdam: Elsevier/North Holland.

Roberts L (1987) Radiation accident grips Goiania. *Science* **238:** 1028–1032.

Rubin P & Casarett GW (1968) *Radiation Syndromes in Clinical Radiation Pathology*, vol. 2. Philadelphia: WB Saunders.

Saenger EL (1986) Radiation accidents. *Annals of Emergency Medicine* **9** 1061-1066.

Sagstuen E, Theisen H & Henriksen T (1983) Dosimetry by ESR spectroscopy following a radiation accident. *Health Physics* **45:** 961–968.

Saral R, Burns WH, Laskin OL, Santos GW & Lietman PS (1981) Acyclovir prophylaxis of herpes simplex virus infections. A randomized double blind controlled trial in bone marrow transplant patients. *New England Journal of Medicine* **305:** 63–67.

Schlein B (1983) *Preparedness and Response in Radiation Accidents*, pp 180–195. Olney, Maryland: US Dept of Health and Human Services Nucleon Lecturn.

Solomon F & Marston RQ (1986) *Medical Implications of Nuclear War*. Washington, DC: National Academy Press.

Stern PJ (1980) Surgical approaches to radiation injuries of the hand. In Hubner F & Fry SA (eds) *The Medical Basis of Nuclear Accident Preparedness*, pp 257–263. Amsterdam: Elsevier/North Holland.

Storb R, Weiden PL, Schroeder ML et al (1976) Marrow grafts between canine littermates, homozygous or heterozygous, for lymphocyte defined histocompatibility antigens. *Transplantation* **21:** 299.

Thomas ED, LeBond R, Graham T et al (1970) Marrow infusions in dogs given sublethal or lethal irradiation. *Radiation Research* **41:** 113–124.

Trentin JJ (1959) Graft-marrow-rejection mortality contrasted to homologous disease in irradiated mice receiving homologous bone marrow. *Journal of the National Cancer Institute* **22:** 219–228.

United Nations (1982) *Ionizing Radiation: Sources and Biological Effects. United Nations Scientific Committee on the Effects of Atomic Radiation*. Report to the General Assembly, with annexes (see specifically Annex J), sales no. E.82.IX.8. New York: UN Publication.

United Nations (1985) *Proceedings of the 35th Session of UNSCEAR. Early Effects in Man of High Doses of Radiation*. Report to the United Nations.

US Nuclear Regulatory Commission (1987) *Report on the Accident at the Chernobyl Nuclear Power Station* (NUREG-1250). Springfield, Virginia: National Technical Information Service.

US Office of Technology Assessment (1987) Bone marrow transplantation using unrelated donors: current clinical status and policy issues.

USSR State Committee on the Utilization of Atomic Energy (1986) *The Accident at the Chernobyl Nuclear Power Plant and its Consequences*. Presented at the IAEA experts meeting August 25–29.

Voelz GL (1980) Current approaches to the management of internally contaminated persons. In Hubner KF & Fry SA (eds) *The Medical Basis of Radiation Accident Preparedness*. Amsterdam: Elsevier/North Holland.

Vriesendorp H (1985) Engraftment of hemopoietic cells. In Van Bekkum D & Lowenberg B (eds) *Bone Marrow Transplantation*. Marcel Dekker.

Wald N (1971) Hematological parameters after acute radiation injury. In *Manual on Radiation Hematology*, pp 253–264. Vienna: International Atomic Energy Agency.

Wald N (1983) Diagnosis and therapy of radiation injuries. *Bulletin of the New York Academy of Medicine* **59:** 1129–1138.

Wilson SG (1959) Radiation-induced gastrointestinal death in the monkey. *American Journal of Pathology* **35:** 1233–1251.

Winston DJ, Ho WG, Gale RP & Champlin RE (1986) Prevention and treatment of infection in leukemia patients. In Gale RP (ed.) *Leukemia Therapy*, pp 213–238. Boston: Blackwell.

Yang Y, Ciarletta AB, Temple PA et al (1986) Human IL-3 (multi-CSF): identification by expression cloning of a novel hematopoietic growth factor related to murine IL-3. *Cell* **47:** 3–10.

6

Growth factors in haemopoiesis

ALISON L. JONES
JOHN L. MILLAR

It has been postulated since 1906 (Carnot and Deflandre, 1906), and shown since the early 1950s (Reissman, 1950; Erslev, 1953) that erythropoiesis is under the control of a humoral factor. Since the mid 1960s in vitro haemopoiesis (initially granulocyte and macrophage colony formation) has been demonstrable, provided a source of exogenous growth factor is added to the culture. The investigation of haemopoiesis in vitro (Dexter, 1984; Metcalf, 1984) has provided the means whereby the factors involved have been isolated and characterized. The availability of recombinant material has provided sufficient quantities of these factors for in vivo testing.

The effects of these factors in vitro have been extensively reviewed elsewhere (Burgess, 1985; Metcalf, 1986; Dexter and Moore, 1986). The purpose of this article is to present the most recent data on their effects in vivo with particular reference to clinical applications. As several of the factors have only recently been identified, their prospective value will be inferred from their in vitro actions.

Erythropoietin is recognized as the main humoral factor involved in the regulation of erythropoiesis. The hunt for a corresponding granulopoietin has been on for some time. In the mid 1960s two groups developed the techniques of growing bone marrow cells in vitro as colonies (Pluznik and Sachs, 1965; Bradley and Metcalf, 1966) and this permitted studies of the relationships between different cell types and their growth requirements. It is now accepted that mature white blood cells arise from multipotent stem cells via inter-mediate cells, and are classified according to their lineage. The earliest progenitors, or stem cells, undergo self-renewal, so maintaining a pool of stem cells. Some stem cells undergo differentiation to committed progenitors of the erythroid, myeloid, megakaryocytic and lymphoid lineages. Sub-sequent maturation of these committed progenitors finally generates the functional end cells. It is likely that there are several regulatory steps in this maturation and so the concept of a single granulopoietin is not realistic.

The colonies of haemopoietic cells require soluble factors for survival and to allow proliferation and differentiation. A family of four main colony-stimulating factors (CSFs) has been identified. These were originally derived from conditioned media (Metcalf, 1986). They have been shown to stimulate precursor cells to form colonies of progeny in vitro and are named

Table 1. The effect of haemopoietic growth factors in vitro and in vivo.

Growth factor	Species	Alternative names	Mol wt	Found in vivo	Main effects	
					in vitro	in vivo*
Erythropoietin (EPO)	murine	none	39000	yes	Formation of erythroid colonies	Stimulates committed erythroid precursors to form erythroblasts: physiological regulator
	human	none	34000	yes		
Granulocyte/macrophage colony-stimulating factor (GM-CSF)	murine	MGI-IGM	23000	yes	Formation of granulocyte/macrophage colonies	Stimulates proliferation and differentiation of committed myelomonocytic precursors Neutrophil activation
	human	CSF-α	30000	yes		
Granulocyte colony-stimulating factor (G-CSF)	murine	MGI-IG	25000	yes	Formation of granulocyte colonies	Stimulates neutrophil production in neutropenic mice
	human	CSF-β	30000	yes		May stimulate neutrophil production in man
Macrophage colony-stimulating factor (M-CSF)	murine	CSF-I, MGI-IM	70000	?	Formation of macrophage colonies	
	human		40000			
Interleukin 3 (IL-3)	murine	multi-CSF, CSF 2 pluripoietin	23000	no	Maintenance and proliferation of CFU and precursors of granulocytes, macrophages, megakaryocytes, eosinophils, mast cells and erythroid cells	Stimulation of CFU, local production of macrophages and granulocytes
	human	none				Induces leukocytosis/eosinophilia in primates
Interleukin 1 (IL-1)	murine	lymphocyte activating factor (LAF) haemopoietin 1 (H-1)	17000	yes	Proliferation of mouse thymocytes Modulates haemopoietic progenitor cells to respond to lineage-restricted factors Induction of IL-2	Radioprotects haemopoietic stem cells, fever, release of acute phase proteins, induction of GM-CSF, IFN
	human					

Factor	Species	Other names	MW	Administration*	Action	Effect on haemopoiesis
Interleukin 2 (IL-2)	murine	TCGF	15 000	no	Expands lymphocyte populations e.g. LAK cells	Needed to promote LAK cell action
	human					
Interleukin 4 (IL-4)	murine	BSF1	20 000	not yet	B cell activation, increases IgG and IgE production, proliferation of T helper cells	Unknown
	human					
Interleukin-5 (IL-5)	murine	EDF	32–62 000	not yet	Stimulates eosinophil production	Unknown
	human		30 000	not yet		
Interleukin-6 (IL-6)	murine	hybridoma growth factor BSF-2, IFN-β2	23–27 000	not yet	Promotes growth of hybridomas and plasmacytomas	Unknown
	human	IFN-β2, BCDF, HGF	26 000	not yet	Stimulates Ig-secretion in B cells Growth of hybridomas and plasmacytomas	Unknown
Tumour necrosis factor (TNF)	murine	lymphotoxin	45 000	yes	Cytotoxic to some tumour cells	No effect on normal haemopoietic cells
	human	cachectin		yes	As above	Produces mild leukocytosis at low dose and transient leukopenia at higher doses
Interferon γ (IFN γ)	murine	immune interferon	40 000	yes	Inhibits normal and malignant haemopoietic cells and activates macrophages	Antitumour effect especially in combination with TNF
	human			yes		

* Exogenous administration (only erythropoietin is a proven physiological regulator).
CFU = colony forming units; LAK = lymphocyte-activated killer cells.

according to their dominant progeny (Dexter and Moore, 1986); hence GM-CSF (granulocyte and macrophage), G-CSF (granulocyte), M-CSF (macrophage) and multi-CSF (now termed interleukin 3; IL-3) which stimulates both lineages via very early progenitor cells. It is now recognized that GM-CSF and IL-3 can also affect erythroid and possibly megakaryocyte development. Other factors which influence the haemopoietic system include the interleukins; IL-1, IL-2, IL-4, IL-5 and IL-6; tumour necrosis factor (TNF); the interferons, IFN α, β and γ, and also factors involved in platelet production. For a glossary of terms see Table 1.

There are potential problems in studying in vivo effects of factors produced and detected in vitro. Early work used factors derived from conditioned media. Retrospectively this presented difficulties in interpretation of results because of contamination with other proteins (and hence possibly other factors; Stone-Wolff et al, 1984), and also with endotoxin which itself results in a temporary neutrophilia. With advances in molecular biology and recombinant DNA technology, sufficient quantities of purified individual factors have been obtained for in vivo testing. However a number of problems still remain.

One problem arises because not all the growth factors can be detected in vivo. This raises the question of whether they have a physiological role which may be enhanced by exogenous administration, or whether they are in vitro artifacts which can be used as pharmacological agents.

CSF (Myers and Robinson, 1975), IL-1 (Kluger et al, 1985) and erythropoietin (Miyake et al, 1977) can all be detected in man. However, IL-2, IL-3 and more recently IL-4, IL-5 and IL-6 have only been found in vitro, although receptors for IL-2 can be detected in man (Greene et al, 1986). IL-2 and IL-3 have effects on haemopoiesis when administered as described below.

It is unclear why these factors have not been detected in vivo. They may only act locally in the haemopoietic tissue and therefore not be detected in plasma. Alternatively they may be produced in very small amounts and cleared rapidly. Certainly, the plasma half-lives of injected factors are short, e.g. that of recombinant IL-3 in mice is between 7 and 10 min (Lord et al, 1986). The plasma half-life may also depend on the route of administration (Mayer et al, 1987). This implies that pharmacokinetic studies will be necessary to determine optimal administration if factors are to be used therapeutically. It is likely that long exposure will be required between factors and target cells, so constant infusion regimes may be necessary (Dexter, 1986). It may also be useful to establish marrow receptor saturation for a given factor to determine the optimal dose and to demonstrate whether factors in plasma have access to the relevant cells in the marrow (Shadduck and Waheed, 1986).

Second, the source of factor may be important. For example, the activity of erythropoietin in vivo is dependent on the protein being highly glycosylated (Erslev, 1987). Growth factors cloned from bacteria are poorly glycosylated, whereas those cloned from mammalian cells preserve glycosylation, and such glycosylation may be relevant to function in vivo. The in vivo action of other factors, e.g. GM-CSF (Mayer et al, 1987), IFN-α (Bose and Hickman, 1977) and IL-2 (Robb and Smith, 1981) does not appear to depend on glycosylation. These variations in activity may be due to differences in clearance mechanisms: erythropoietin undergoes hepatic clearance (Neufeld and Ashwell, 1980) whereas GM-CSF, IL-2 and IFN-α undergo renal clearance (Bino et al, 1982). Other structural features are important for biological activity, for example reduction of disulphide bonds in M-CSF eliminates its biological activity (Das and Stanley, 1982). Initial testing in vivo should be done with native and cloned products to establish that they have similar activity.

Third, there is evidence that many of the factors are multifunctional. IL-1, for example, stimulates thymocyte proliferation (Gery et al, 1972; Oppenheim et al, 1986), acts on the liver to release acute-phase proteins, on synovial fibroblasts with collagenase production and as an endogenous pyrogen (Dinarello, 1986b). When IL-2 is used pharmacologically, it has adverse effects on vascular permeability and hepatorenal function (Lotze et al, 1986). It is likely therefore that the in vivo use of some of the factors may be limited by unacceptable side-effects.

There is a complex inter-relationship between the factors, which makes analysis of individual actions difficult (Balkwill and Smyth, 1987). A factor may induce release of others from intermediate cells: this is the so-called lymphokine cascade (Dexter, 1986). In combination, factors may have additive or synergistic interactions, and individual factors may modify receptors for others. Therefore it is difficult to attribute an effect in vivo to any one particular factor and indeed combinations may be necessary for best effects.

The potential uses of haemopoietic growth factors lie in four main areas. Firstly, they can be used to stimulate recovery of normal haemopoiesis, in particular white cells. Second, some factors may enhance functional activity of neutrophils. This could be useful in bone marrow transplantation and also in refractory infection. Third, they may have a therapeutic role either by direct tumour cell killing or by mediating the release of other cytotoxic products. Fourth, they may prove useful in the treatment of leukaemia by inducing differentiation of leukaemic cells to functional end cells.

ERYTHROPOIESIS

Erythropoietin represents a good example of the ability of factors to correct haemopoiesis. It has been known for some time that exogenous erythropoietin can be used to correct the red cell volume in animals which had been rendered anaemic by nephrectomy (e.g. Anagnostou et al, 1977). This work has recently been extended to man. In patients with end-stage renal disease maintained on haemodialysis, erythropoietin administration improved both the patients' haemoglobin concentration and general well-being (Winearls et al, 1986; Eschbach et al, 1987). Recombinant human erythropoietin was administered three times a week as a bolus after dialysis, with an escalating dose schedule ranging from 3 to 192 IU/kg. A rise in haemoglobin concentration from 6.1 g/dl (range 4.6–8.8) to 10.3 g/dl (9.5–12.8) was observed in

9/10 patients and these patients were no longer transfusion-dependent (Winearls et al, 1986).

Anaemia in renal disease is associated with low endogenous erythro-poietin levels. It is still not clear if exogenous erythropoietin therapy could benefit patients with anaemia in whom endogenous erythropoietin levels are normal or high. Indeed, some patients with aplastic anaemia have high endogenous levels of erythropoietin, and therefore further increases have little value. In some haemoglobinopathies (e.g. sickle cell disease and thalassaemias) an increase in haematocrit may actually be dangerous because of increased viscosity and the risks of thrombosis. Such compli-cations have been seen in renal patients—two with blocked fistulae and one other patient experiencing an episode of hypertensive encephalopathy (Winearls et al, 1986). Erythropoietin therapy is associated with a fall in serum ferritin. Although this could be useful in anaemic patients with iron overload, it is important to ensure that patients have adequate supplies of iron and other haematinics during therapy to avoid developing deficiencies that might compromise their response.

Erythropoietin could also be used for short-term stimulation of bone marrow prior to venesection of blood for elective autologous transfusion (Surgenor, 1987).

Other factors may be necessary for the optimal effect of erythropoietin. For example, the lymphokine IL-3 has been shown to increase the number of cells capable of differentiating into erythroblasts in the presence of erythropoietin (Goldwasser et al, 1983). Androgens also appear to sensitize the cells committed to erythroid differentiation to the effects of erythro-poietin (Neff et al, 1981).

COLONY-STIMULATING FACTORS

There is some evidence that CSFs regulate haemopoiesis in vivo. GM-CSF has been detected in normal mouse serum (Robinson et al, 1967) and in human serum and urine (Myers and Robinson, 1975). Also the levels of CSF increase in response to infection and, in mice, to bacterial products such as endotoxin (Burgess, 1985). Levels are elevated in serum and urine of some patients with myeloid leukaemia (Metcalf et al, 1971) and with aplastic anaemia (Gordon-Smith, personal communication). Some human tumours synthesize CSF constitutively and are associated with neutrophilia in man; they result in neutrophilia when transplanted as xenografts in immune-deficient mice (Okabe et al, 1978).

Early experiments on mice used CSF derived from mouse embryo extract (Bradley et al, 1969) or human urine (Metcalf and Stanley, 1971). The results suggested that it might be possible to manipulate granulopoiesis in vivo. More recently, recombinant GM-CSF has been tested in rodents and primates. There was an increase in end-cells (neutrophils, macrophages and eosinophils) in the peritoneal cavity of adult mice injected intraperitoneally with murine recombinant GM-CSF (rmGM-CSF; Metcalf et al, 1987a). The dose ranged from 6–200 ng per mouse and the response was dose-related.

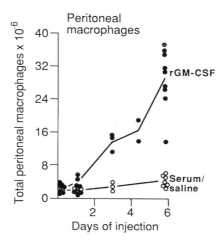

Figure 1. Progressive rise in total peritoneal macrophages in C57BL mice injected three times daily with 200 ng rGM-CSF or 0.2 ml mouse serum/saline. Each point represents an individual mouse. From Metcalf et al (1987a), with permission.

The cells showing the best response were peritoneal macrophages in animals given 200 ng rmGM-CSF t.d.s. for 6 days (Figure 1). Although there was a modest increase in the numbers of granulocyte-macrophage progenitors in the spleen, there was a decrease in progenitor cells in the bone marrow with a net decrease in progenitors, suggesting that differentiation and maturation had occurred at the expense of progenitor cell self-renewal.

In vivo experiments have also utilized the growth factor G-CSF which stimulates only neutrophil production. Unlike the other CSFs, human G-CSF is active in mice. Using G-CSF purified from medium conditioned by a human bladder carcinoma cell line (5637), it has been demonstrated that the number of peripheral neutrophils can be increased eightfold in mice injected for 15 days (Tamura et al, 1987). Purified murine CSF-1 (M-CSF) had no consistent effect when administered to mice (Shadduck et al, 1987) although relatively few marrow receptors were saturated at the doses used.

Donahue et al (1986) have demonstrated a substantial leukocytosis and reticulocytosis, associated with bone marrow hyperplasia, in primates given continuous i.v. infusion of human rGM-CSF ($50 \, U \, kg^{-1} \, min^{-1}$) over 10 days. The rise started after 1–3 days and was dependent on the continued presence of GM-CSF with counts falling to near pretreatment levels within a few days of discontinuation of therapy (Figure 2). This suggests that GM-CSF does not act at the stem cell level, but enhances the proliferation of a committed progenitor with limited self-renewal. After the stimulus has gone the effect is short-lived. No substantial ill-effects were seen, although some animals developed antibodies to human GM-CSF. It is not yet known if such antibodies would compromise further therapy. The effects were greatest in the eosinophil count (30-fold increase). A similar effect has been seen in a virus-infected, pancytopenic monkey but again only for the duration of treatment. In this instance the dose was increased to

$500\,\mathrm{U\,kg^{-1}\,min^{-1}}$ and the duration of therapy shortened to 7 days (Figure 2). The pancytopenic monkey had high endogenous erythropoietin levels. The increased reticulocytosis in this animal was greater than in the healthy animals, suggesting there may have been a synergistic interaction between erythropoietin and GM-CSF, enhancing erythropoiesis. Another group has confirmed these findings but has not seen effects on erythrocyte or platelet counts in treated healthy monkeys (Mayer et al, 1987). They also noted that the subcutaneous route administered thrice daily was more effective than a 6 h i.v. infusion daily over a 7-day period. The subcutaneous route may improve the bioavailability of GM-CSF.

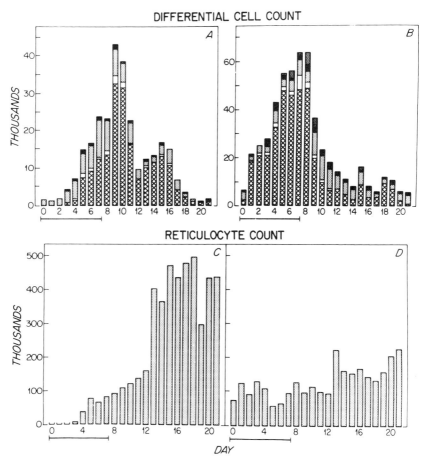

Figure 2. Serial differential counts (A,B) and reticulocyte (C,D) counts of a pancytopenic rhesus monkey (A,C) and a healthy rhesus monkey (B,D) continuously infused with recombinant human GM-CSF for 7 days. From Donahue et al (1986), with permission. ▨ Eosinophils; ■ Monocytes; ▒ Lymphocytes; ☐ Bands; ▩ Neutrophils.

These in vivo effects have generated interest in using CSFs therapeutically to enhance reconstitution of haemopoiesis after chemotherapy, radiotherapy or bone marrow transplantation. With recombinant G-CSF, Shimamura et al (1987) restored granulopoiesis in mice with bone marrow damaged by 5-fluorouracil (5-FU). Daily administration of 10^5 U per mouse per day restored the neutrophil count to normal after 12 days, whereas in animals not receiving G-CSF, the neutrophil count at this time was still less than 10% of normal. Welte and co-workers damaged the bone marrow of primates with cyclophosphamide (Welte et al, 1987a), total body irradiation (TBI), or busulphan (Welte et al, 1987b) and attempted to restore granulopoiesis with rhG-CSF. Of the three monkeys receiving cyclophosphamide the most effective restoration of granulopoiesis was seen when G-CSF was administered both before and after cyclophosphamide, although significant shortening of neutropenia was also seen when G-CSF was given only after cyclophosphamide. The period of neutropenia after autologous bone marrow transplantation in monkeys conditioned with 10 Gy TBI was shortened by the administration of rhG-CSF at either 50 or 100 µg kg^{-1} day^{-1}. Furthermore, the post bone marrow transplantation absolute neutrophil count could be maintained for 3 months by the daily administration of G-CSF (Welte et al, 1987b). GM-CSF has been used to accelerate neutrophil recovery following autologous bone marrow transplantation in primates whose bone marrow had been ablated by TBI (Nienhuis et al, 1987). The factor was given by continuous i.v. infusion at 50 U kg^{-1} min^{-1} either both before and after transplantation or only after transplantation. Neutrophil recovery to 1.0×10^9/l was reached at 8–9 days post-transplant in treated animals, compared with 17 or 24 days for the two control animals. The counts fell to those of control animals after discontinuation of GM-CSF. Accelerated platelet recovery was seen in four out of the five treated animals. Two animals developed oedema, diarrhoea and hypoalbuminaemia which resolved with supportive care after discontinuing GM-CSF. Marrow engraftment was not compromised by GM-CSF.

The rise in peripheral white blood count in these studies was largely a result of an increase in neutrophils. This rise was early, suggesting that the CSF caused release of neutrophils into the circulation. However, the rise could also be sustained over long periods; Donahue et al (1986) treated one monkey for 21 days. The maintenance of elevated neutrophil counts coupled with the observed normal (Mayer et al, 1987) or increased (Donahue et al, 1986) cellularity of the bone marrow suggested that the factor was having an effect on both neutrophil maturation and release.

The prompt response of neutrophils to CSF is similar to the rapid response in normal hosts to infection (Marsh et al, 1967). There is in vitro evidence to show that CSFs enhance mature neutrophil function. Human GM-CSF has been demonstrated to inhibit neutrophil migration (Gasson et al, 1984) and to stimulate the functional activity of mature granulocytes and macrophages (Metcalf, 1986). Further research in vitro (Fleischmann et al, 1986) showed that CSFs enhanced phagocytosis of bacteria by human neutrophils.

Matsumoto et al (1987) have demonstrated in vivo enhancement of resistance to bacterial challenge in neutropenic mice by the administration of human G-CSF. Mayer and colleagues demonstrated enhanced neutrophil function in vivo in primates treated with GM-CSF with increased oxidative metabolism, as measured by generation of a superoxide anion and by enhanced antibacterial activity (Mayer et al, 1987). Indirect evidence for a role for CSFs in combating infection is the elevation of endogenous CSFs in post-endotoxic sera (Burgess, 1985). In mice intraperitoneal injection of GM-CSF produced an accumulation of neutrophils in the peritoneal cavity (Metcalf et al, 1987a). This raises the possibility of using CSFs as local agents in combating infection.

The leukocytosis and enhanced neutrophil function induced by CSFs suggest a variety of potential applications in man. The restoration of haemo-poiesis in idiopathic or iatrogenic myelosuppression and the treatment of refractory infection in normal or immunocompromised patients are areas for consideration. It is uncertain whether GM-CSF or G-CSF will have the greater use. However, as myeloid leukaemic blasts possess receptors for GM-CSF (Metcalf, 1986), the use of this factor in patients with myeloid leukaemia may be inadvisable.

As this is a new area of therapy, data from clinical trials are limited. Partially purified human urinary CSF has been used in patients undergoing chemotherapy (Motoyshi et al, 1986) and in patients undergoing bone marrow transplantation (Masaoka et al, 1986). These studies suggested some benefit in terms of neutrophil recovery. However recombinant human GM-CSF has superseded this source of GM-CSF. Groopman et al (1987) administered rhGM-CSF to 16 patients with acquired immunodeficiency syndrome (AIDS) with leukopenia. A dose-dependent increase in circulat-ing leukocytes was observed with a maximal count ranging from 4575 ($\pm$ 2397) cells/μl at a dose of 1.3×10^3 U kg^{-1} day^{-1} to 48 700 cells/μl in the patient receiving the highest dose (2.0×10^4 U kg^{-1} day^{-1}). Each patient received a single i.v. dose, then 48 h later a 14-day continuous infusion. No life-threatening toxicity was observed, although some patients exhibited low-grade fever, myalgia, phlebitis and flushing.

A small study using rhG-CSF in patients undergoing chemotherapy suggested a higher neutrophil recovery at day 14 (Gabrilove et al, 1987). In another study rhG-CSF was administered to patients with small cell lung cancer (Hernandez Bronchud et al, 1987). G-CSF was given as a continuous infusion over 5 days to 11 patients in a phase 1 study, and a maximal response in peripheral neutrophils was seen at doses of 5–10 μg kg^{-1} day^{-1}. These neutrophils were functionally competent in tests of motility and bactericidal activity. In a phase 2 study G-CSF was given to the same patients for 14 days on alternate cycles of chemotherapy with a median of 80% reduction in absolute neutrophilia and a significant protection against infective episodes.

The enhancement of neutrophil numbers appeared to last only for the duration of CSF therapy. This may be an important consideration in employing these factors in therapy. However, there is no evidence as yet of tachyphylaxis, so administration may be feasible over a long time period. The most likely use will be in enhancing neutrophil number and function in the short term, especially during infection. Initial results in man appear to parallel the animal data as reported.

INTERLEUKIN 3

IL-3 was originally derived from the murine myelomonocytic cell line WEHI 3 (Ihle et al, 1982) and is also known as multi-CSF (Table 1). It is predominantly a product of activated T-cells. In view of its actions it is convenient to consider IL-3 in conjunction with the CSFs. In vitro IL-3 has a wider field of action than the other CSFs as it stimulates both multipotent and committed myeloid progenitors (Dexter and Moore, 1986). Moreover, the evidence suggests that IL-3 does not support self-renewal of stem cells, but rather very early progenitor cells which become responsive to IL-3 and are then committed to differentiation. These cells may subsequently become responsive to GM-CSF. In vitro, IL-3 can support the growth of cells which generate spleen colony-forming units (CFU-S), thought to represent the haemopoietic stem cells in mice, but cannot do so indefinitely (Spivak et al, 1985). The development of maturation markers and the ability to respond to GM-CSF suggest that IL-3 induces differentiation in the target cells (Ihle, 1986). In addition, IL-3 has been shown to increase the number of cells which can differentiate in response to erythropoietin (Goldwasser et al, 1983).

In vitro there is evidence for interaction between IL-3 and other factors. For example, Bertoncello et al (1986) demonstrated synergy between CSF-1 and IL-3. Using factors derived from conditioned media they produced progenitors with high proliferative potential (HPP) in agar, not seen when

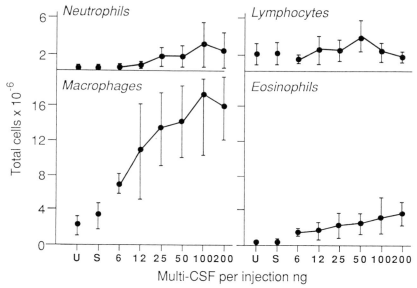

Figure 3. Rises in absolute numbers of peritoneal macrophages, neutrophils, and eosinophils in BALB/c mice after injection for 6 days of various concentrations of rmulti-CSF. U = untreated mice; S = mice injected with 0.2 ml of carrier-mouse serum/saline. From Metcalf et al (1987b), with permission.

either factor was used alone. For a recent review of these and other in vitro findings see Quesenberry (1986).

IL-3 has not been described as occurring in vivo in normal, stressed or malignant haemopoiesis although in vitro IL-3-dependent lines have been established from retrovirus-induced murine leukaemias and lymphomas (Dexter et al, 1980; Greenberger et al, 1983). While the effects of exogenous recombinant murine IL-3 have been investigated in mice, the human equivalent has only recently been identified and cloned (Wong et al, 1985).

Intraperitoneal administration of rmIL-3 in mice resulted in a dose-dependent local increase in neutrophils, eosinophils and macrophages, an increase in splenic weight and mast cell content (Figure 3) but little effect on bone marrow or peripheral blood count (Metcalf et al, 1987b). This contrasted with the administration of rmGM-CSF which resulted in a net decrease in progenitor cells through marrow depletion and which also did not affect mast cell precursors in the spleen. Multipotent stem cells, as

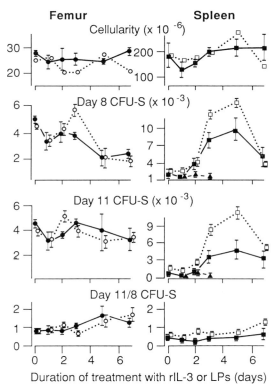

Figure 4. Changes in cellularity and spleen colony forming units (CFU-S) in mice treated by chronic infusion of rIL-3 or lipopolysaccharide (LPS).
Bone marrow cells: rIL-3 ●; LPS (50 ng/h) ○.
Spleen cells: rIL-3 ■; LPS (50 ng/h) □;
                          LPS (10 fg/h) ▲.
From Lord et al (1986), with permission.

measured by CFU-S, increased in number following administration of IL-3 in vivo (Figure 4; Lord et al, 1986). These results were similar to those obtained using endotoxin in the form of lipopolysaccharide. Similar results using continuous subcutaneous administration were noted by Kindler et al (1986), who also demonstrated that IL-3 could compensate for the expected reduction in haemopoietic activity following sublethal irradiation. In these experiments progenitor cells were increased in the spleen but were reduced in bone marrow. The erythroid lineage was stimulated, suggesting that IL-3 may either directly stimulate erythropoiesis in vivo or may act in concert with another haemopoietic growth factor, possibly erythropoietin.

IL-3 can support the growth of blast cells in vitro (Sonoda et al, 1988) which may be a caveat to its ultimate use in man. Studies in primates (Yang et al, 1987) show a modest leukocytosis when IL-3 is administered by continuous infusion, comparable with low-dose GM-CSF administration but with delayed kinetics. Eosinophilia and, in some animals, a marked increase in platelet count were observed. If the monkeys were treated with IL-3 prior to very low-dose GM-CSF infusion, a rapid, very marked leuko-cytosis was observed, suggesting a synergistic interaction.

INTERLEUKIN 1 AND TUMOUR NECROSIS FACTOR

Other factors have been implicated in the regulation of haemopoiesis; these act in conjunction with CSFs to enhance the proliferative response in vitro (Stanley et al, 1986). These factors appear to modulate early progenitor cells to respond to factors which would normally act on more differentiated cells. One such factor, haemopoietin 1 (H1), has been purified from medium conditioned by a human bladder tumour cell line (Jubinsky and Stanley, 1985). It was shown to enhance CSF-1 (M-CSF) stimulation of macrophage colony formation in vitro. H1 is now known to be interleukin 1 (IL-1; Mochizuki et al, 1987). Stem cells cultured with IL-1 and M-CSF produce colonies containing mature macrophages, although neither factor can support stem cell survival and differentiation alone (Dexter, personal communication). Similar synergy is seen between IL-1 and GM-CSF or IL-3.

IL-1 has synergistic effects with factors other than CSFs. In vitro, IL-1 shows enhanced tumour cell killing in conjunction with IFNγ or with TNF (Ruggiero and Baglioni, 1987).

IL-1 is mainly produced by activated macrophages but represents a family of molecules which can be produced by a variety of other cells, including some human B-cell lines (Scala et al, 1984), and keratinocytes (Bell et al, 1987). Its production by thymic epithelial cells has been reported (Le et al, 1987) although this may be an indirect effect (Mizutani et al, 1987). Monocytes produce two major forms which differ on isoelectric focusing: IL-1β with a pI value of 7 and IL-1α with a pI value of 5. IL-1β is responsible for most of the biological activity in man (Oppenheim et al, 1986). IL-1 activity has been detected in vivo in mice (Gahring et al, 1984) and in man (Bendtzen et al, 1984). The variety of tissues producing IL-1 and indeed, possessing receptors for IL-1 may suggest that it can modulate growth in tissues other than the haemopoietic system.

In vitro IL-1 is necessary for the production of IL-2 from activated T-cells as well as being essential in T-cell clonal expansion. It is implicated in the production of IFNγ and GM-CSF from T-cells in vitro (Oppenheim et al, 1986).

In vivo, exogenous administration of IL-1 to mice results in high serum GM-CSF at 3 and 6 h after injection (Vogel et al, 1987) but IFNγ was not detected. Synergy between IL-1 and CSFs may also exist in vivo. A combination of IL-1 and G-CSF enhanced haemopoietic recovery, measured by CFU-S in mice given 5-fluorouracil (5-FU) (Moore and Warren, 1987). IL-1 protects haemopoietic tissue in mice from radiation damage (Neta et al, 1986). Protection is most effective when IL-1 is given 20 h before irradiation and this effect may be enhanced by the addition of TNF (Neta et al, 1987).

IL-1 is an early mediator of the acute-phase response to inflammation and immunostimulation (Dinarello, 1986b). Exogenous IL-1 produces fever in animals (Dinarello, 1986a) and endogenous IL-1 has also been detected in man during fever (Bendtzen et al, 1984). IL-1 stimulates release of the prostaglandin E series from macrophages, fibroblasts, skeletal muscle and chondrocytes as well as from hypothalamic and cortical cells (Dinarello, 1986b).

TNF has similarities with IL-1 in its effects. It too, induces fever, hepatic acute-phase protein synthesis and collagenase in synovial cells. However TNF does not activate T-cells, although it can induce GM-CSF production (Munker et al, 1986).

TNF is a polypeptide mediator which exists in two forms—TNFα produced by macrophages (cachectin), and TNFβ produced by lymphocytes (lymphotoxin). While most of the clinical interest in TNF is centred around its possible role as an anticancer agent (Blick et al, 1987) and also as a mediator of cachexia (Beutler and Cerami, 1986), experiments suggest that it also has effects on the haemopoietic system. It may act as a differentiating agent on myeloid cells in vitro (Takeda et al, 1986). In man, administration of TNF in a single dose caused transient neutrophilia but prolonged administration results both in leukopenia and thrombocytopenia (Selby et al, 1988).

Combinations of TNF with IFNγ have enhanced cytotoxicity against murine tumours (Brouckaert et al, 1986) and human tumours grown as xenografts in immune-deprived mice (Balkwill et al, 1987). TNF and IL-1 also show enhanced cytotoxicity against tumour cells in vitro (Ruggiero and Baglioni, 1987).

INTERLEUKIN 2

IL-2, originally called T-cell growth factor, is a polypeptide (molecular weight 12 000) secreted mainly by helper T-cells, although all T-cell subsets can produce it (Pfizenmaier et al, 1984). The major role of IL-2 is the clonal expansion of antigen-reactive T-cells of all classes, whose IL-2 receptors have been induced and activated by antigen or mitogen (Bonnard et al, 1979). The initial activation is dependent on the presence of IL-1. Although T-cell proliferation in vitro has an absolute requirement for IL-2, endogenous IL-2 has not been detected in vivo. However, using monoclonal antibodies, a soluble form of the IL-2 receptor (IL-2R) can be detected in man (Greene et al, 1986). This has been detected in peripheral blood from normal adults so its significance in disease is not clear.

IL-2 induces the secretion of IFNγ by T-cells (Farrar et al, 1981), enhances natural killer (NK) cell activity (Henney et al, 1981) and activates lymphocyte killing in vitro.

Yron et al (1980) demonstrated that the incubation of human peripheral blood lymphocytes or murine spleen cells with IL-2 resulted in the generation of cells with the capacity to lyse fresh syngeneic or autologous tumour cells. These lymphocyte-activated killer (LAK) cells lyse tumour cells but not normal cells. Mazumber and Rosenberg subsequently showed regression of established pulmonary melanoma metastases in mice by the intravenous infusion of IL-2 with LAK cells generated from autologous murine lymphocytes expanded in vitro (Mazumber and Rosenberg, 1984). A similar result could be shown by infusing a high dose of rIL-2 alone, which was shown to generate endogenous LAK cells in situ in mouse spleen (Rosenberg et al, 1985).

This work has been extended to patients with advanced cancer. Patients were treated with rIL-2, either by bolus or by continuous infusion, together with autologous LAK cells which had previously been harvested by leuko-phoresis and expanded in vitro by incubation with IL-2. The continued presence of IL-2 was necessary for the maintenance of the LAK cells. Rosenberg et al (1987) reported on 106 patients receiving IL-2 and LAK cells and on 46 patients receiving IL-2 alone. Although only a small number of patients showed a response, some of these responses were substantial in cancers which are normally resistant to therapy. The remissions were transient, lasting a maximum of a few months.

The toxicity of such treatment was considerable and severe side-effects were attributed to the IL-2 administration rather than the LAK cell infusion. Patients experienced fever, malaise, nausea, vomiting and diarrhoea which abated when the IL-2 infusion was discontinued. Most patients had hepatic dysfunction with raised bilirubin and some experienced transient neuro-psychiatric disturbances. Transient cardiac arrhythmias were observed and myocardial infarction was diagnosed in four patients. Most patients exhibited haemopoietic suppression and transfusions were required in 150 out of 180 courses. A smaller number of patients exhibited thrombocytopenia and/or neutropenia. Therapy with continuous infusion of IL-2 as opposed to bolus administration appears to be less toxic (West et al, 1987).

Further attempts to reduce toxicity are being made. One possibility is the use of IL-2 without LAK cells (West et al, 1987). Another is the combination of such therapy at lower doses with other agents, either other biological factors or conventional cytotoxic drugs. Regional administration may be possible (Lotzova, 1986). So far the use of IL-2 and LAK cells in man has been confined to patients with advanced and bulky disease. Animal data suggest that anticancer therapy using biological agents is more effective when employed against small disease volumes (Balkwill, 1985) over long time periods, and this may also prove true for IL-2.

It is not yet clear whether the presence of LAK cells is necessary for the efficacy of IL-2 or indeed, if so, whether lymphocytes or NK cells are the optimal cells for expansion. A more recent approach to reducing the need for large numbers of LAK cells and high-dose IL-2 infusions and hence toxicity has been to expand tumour-infiltrating lymphocytes in vitro with IL-2 (Rosenberg et al, 1986). In mice these cells were 50 to 100 times more effective than LAK cells and had activity against tumours which did not respond to LAK cell therapy. Also these tumour-infiltrating lymphocytes mediated an antitumour effect in the absence of IL-2, although their activity was optimal in its presence. This combination was further enhanced by the administration of conventional chemotherapy, in this instance cyclophosphamide.

FACTORS AFFECTING B-CELLS

Another function of IL-2 is the activation and differentiation of B-cells to mature immunoglobulin-secreting plasma cells, both indirectly by inducing B cell growth and differentiation factors, and by the direct support of B cells with IL-2 receptors (Dexter and Moore, 1986). B cell development and function does not depend solely on IL-2 but on a complex interplay of factors, including IL-4, IL-5, IL-6 and IFNγ.

Interleukin 4

IL-4 is produced by activated T-cells and so far its activity has been tested in vitro only. It was originally thought to be a B cell-specific growth factor (BSF1), but now it is recognized to be less specific. Both murine and human forms of this glycoprotein have been identified. IL-4 has a role in B cell activation (transition from G_0 to G_1 in the cell cycle), co-stimulation (in conjunction with other B-cell activators), B cell division and differentiation (Abbas, 1987). It enhances IgG1 (Noma et al, 1986) and IgE (Coffman and Carty, 1986) production by B cells and can also cause proliferation of mast cell lines (Smith and Rennick, 1986). IL-4 maintains murine macrophages in vitro and increases their antigen-presenting ability (Zlotnik et al, 1987a). IL-4 also stimulates the proliferation of human helper T cells in vitro (Yokota et al, 1986). Furthermore, IL-4 seems to have some IL-1-like activity as it can stimulate thymocyte proliferation (Zlotnik et al, 1987b).

Interleukin 5

IL-5 is primarily an eosinophil growth factor. Eosinophilia is T cell-dependent (Basten and Beeson, 1970), which suggests that a soluble factor might be implicated in its control as many of the known growth factors are T cell products. T cell clones derived from mice infected with a parasite (*Mesocestoides corti*) were found to produce a factor which stimulated eosinophil differentiation in murine bone marrow cultures (Sanderson et al, 1985). This factor, now called IL-5, also stimulated human eosinophil colonies in vitro (Lopez et al, 1986). Human IL-5 has been cloned and characterized (Campbell et al, 1987) and is highly lineage-specific so may be involved in the regulation of eosinophilia. GM-CSF and IL-3 can also stimulate eosinophil colonies in vitro as they are multilineage in their effects.

In addition to its effects on eosinophils, murine IL-5 is also a B-cell growth factor. IL-5 has the actions of the factors previously termed B-cell growth factor II (Kinashi et al, 1986) and T cell-replacing factor (TRF; Takatsu et al, 1987). However, no B cell activity has been detected with the recombinant human preparation of IL-5 (Clutterbuck et al, 1987).

Interleukin 6

IL-6 was discovered independently by separate research groups working on haemopoietic cell regulators, hence its variety of names (IFNβ 2, BSF-2 and hybridoma/plasmacytoma growth factor; HPGF; Van Damme, 1987b). Molecular sequencing permitted a clearer characterization of this factor and simplified the nomenclature.

IL-6 is produced by many cell types—fibroblasts, endothelial cells, monocytes, B and T cells and some carcinoma cells. IL-6 is induced by a variety of stimuli—TNF, IL-1 (Van Damme et al, 1987), viruses, platelet-derived growth factor (PDGF), foreign RNA and metabolic inhibitors (Billiau, 1987). The most potent inducer of IL-6 known so far is IL-1, raising the possibility that IL-6 may mediate some of the effects of IL-1.

IL-6 is a B cell differentiation factor for normal B blasts and for Epstein–Barr virus-transformed B cell lines (Hirano et al, 1985) and induces immunoglobulin secretion in response to stimuli. An identical factor is produced by some tumour lines and may be related in vivo to autoimmune conditions associated with some malignant diseases (Hirano et al, 1987). Human IL-6 also allows the in vitro growth of mouse plasmacytomas which can only normally be maintained by in vivo passage (Van Damme et al, 1987). IL-6 was originally described as IFNβ2 but its antiviral action is weak (Van Damme et al, 1987) and it has no similarities with IFNβ1.

Interferons

Interferon γ (IFNγ) is a product of T lymphocytes (Farrar et al, 1981). It has several effects on the haemopoietic and immune systems. In vitro IFNγ inhibits myelopoiesis (Coutinho et al, 1986) and may have inhibitory effects on both normal and malignant cells. This work was done using partially purified IFN, so other factors may have been present and influenced these results (Stone-Wolff et al, 1984). Such interactions can be exploited and more recent work using recombinant material has suggested synergistic interactions between IFNγ and TNF (Brouckaert et al, 1986).

In vitro IFNγ is a macrophage activator (Pace et al, 1983) of murine cells and also augments monocyte cytotoxicity in human cells towards *Leishmania donovani* (Murray et al, 1983). Cloned murine IFNγ stimulates B-cells to produce immunoglobulin (Liebson et al, 1984).

All the IFNs are known to have growth inhibitory actions (Balkwill and Smyth, 1987) in the haemopoietic system. IFNαs have been used in the management of malignant disease in man and are of established value in hairy-cell leukaemia (Quesada et al, 1984). They are also active in chronic myeloid leukaemia (Bergsagel et al, 1986) and some lymphomas, although their role in these and other non-haematological malignancies is less established.

MEGAKARYOCYTE FACTORS

So far we have discussed stimulators of erythropoiesis and granulopoiesis. Humoral factors may be important in the regulation of megakaryocyte and platelet production although research at present is confined to in vitro studies. Platelets develop from megakaryocytes. Two megakaryocyte progenitors are recognized in human bone marrow—the colony forming unit (CFU-MK) and the more primitive burst forming unit (BFU-MK; Hoffman et al, 1987). Factors can act by stimulating the proliferation of progenitor cells and secondly the same, or different, factors can act by accelerating maturation of megakaryocyte cytoplasm before platelet budding (Straneva et al, 1987).

Erythropoietin, GM-CSF and IL-3 (Williams et al, 1984; Quesenberry et al, 1985) have effects at either or both levels in vitro. These factors act directly on cells of megakaryocytic lineage rather than via release of other factors (Hoffman et al, 1987). The number of megakaryocytes in mouse spleens in vivo can be elevated by recombinant human erythropoietin in high doses (McDonald et al, 1987). Increased platelet counts have been seen when IL-3 was infused into primates (Yang et al, 1987).

Specific factors for megakaryocyte development have been identified: megakaryocyte colony-stimulating factor (MK-CSF; Williams et al, 1984), which affects the clonal expansion of megakaryocytes, and a second factor which controls the later stages of megakaryocyte development (Long et al, 1982). Serum from patients with aplastic anaemia (AAS) promotes mega-karyocyte colony formation from normal human bone marrow with both morphologically recognizable megakaryocytes and smaller, earlier platelet glycoprotein (PGP)-positive cells (Hoffman et al, 1981). Purified MK-CSF from AAS stimulates only the smaller cell type. Anti-MK-CSF (produced against purified MK-CSF; Yang et al, 1986) reduces the ability of both AAS and MK-CSF to promote colony formation from normal bone marrow. The stimulation for the production of MK-CSF would seem to be related to MK numbers rather than platelet numbers, as serum from patients with thrombocytopenia but normal or elevated megakaryocytes does not stimu-late MK colonies in vitro (Hoffmann et al, 1981). Terminal differentiation of megakaryocytes may be under the control of separate factors (Straneva et al, 1986) although another group has reported one factor responsible for proliferation of CFU-MK and later stages of megakaryocyte development (Long et al, 1982). Megakaryocyte and platelet growth factors may have some importance as independent regulators of megakaryocytopoiesis but are more likely to form a part of the complicated cytokine network.

ANTIBODIES TO FACTORS AND THEIR RECEPTORS

Antibodies are available to erythropoietin, IL-1, IL-3, G-CSF, M-CSF and GM-CSF and may allow further investigation of the physiological roles of these factors. When antiserum to M-CSF was administered to mice, there was no decrease in either granulopoiesis or monocytopoiesis (Shadduck et al, 1987). However, if the antiserum was administered to mice bearing diffusion chambers there was a decrease in granulopoiesis within the chamber (Shadduck et al, 1986). This may be a result of other factors in vivo which determine the response to CSF or antisera to CSF.

Antibodies to the IL-2 receptor have been used to reverse allograft rejection in cardiac transplants in rats (Kupiec-Weglinski et al, 1986). Exogenous IL-2 could enhance T-cell-mediated graft-versus-host disease (GvHD) in mice which underwent allogeneic bone marrow transplantation (Malkovsky et al, 1987), although IL-2 did not enhance GvHD in T-cell-depleted marrow. It is speculative whether antibodies to IL-2 could be useful in GvHD or whether there could be a role for IL-2 itself in restoring immune function in T-cell-depleted marrow. However, T-cell depletion of marrow, given to patients treated for myeloid leukaemia, is associated with an increased incidence of leukaemic relapse (Apperley et al, 1986), so caution is needed when manipulating T-cell products in man. Mice injected with murine anti-IL-2 fail to mount a cytolytic T-cell response (Granelli-Piperno et al, 1984).

Anti-TNF has been used to reduce acute GvHD in mice (Piguet et al, 1987) although there was no effect on chronic GvHD. Passive immunization against TNF protected mice from lethal endotoxin (Beutler et al, 1985) and this may be possible with anti-TNF antibodies.

GROWTH FACTORS AND DISEASE

Deficient production of factors has been recognized in vitro in the leukocytes of some patients with disease, but this could be artefactual and not reflect the in vivo situation. Reduced IL-2 has been seen in cells from some patients with AIDS, diabetes and autoimmune disease (Gupta, 1986; Kaye et al, 1986). Reduced IFNα has been observed in patients with chronic hepatitis B and myeloproliferative states and has had some use in treating these conditions (Dinarello and Mier, 1987).

APLASTIC ANAEMIA

There are abnormalities of haemopoietic factor production in cells and sera from patients with aplastic anaemia. Increased IL-2 production from peripheral blood lymphocytes and increased expression of the IL-2 receptor have been observed (Gascon et al, 1985). Spontaneous IFNγ production and increased unregulated production of IFNγ following lectin stimulation have also been seen (Zoumbos et al, 1985). Raised IFNγ levels fall during therapy with antithymocyte globulin but no consistent change in IL-2 levels has been seen (Young et al, 1987). IL-1 production by monocytes is lower in aplastic anaemia (Gascon et al, unpublished data). However, increased levels of CSF are detectable in urine and serum from these patients.

These abnormalities cannot be accounted for by multiple transfusion (Young et al, 1987). There may be inhibitory factors which act in aplastic anaemia and there is interest in interferons in this role. As factors form a complex cascade, a derangement in one would be expected to produce others so it is difficult to determine their role in the pathogenesis and possible therapy of aplastic anaemia. Trials are underway using GM-CSF in patients to eradicate refractory infection.

LEUKAEMOGENESIS

CSFs act in vitro to allow limited self-renewal of progenitor cells and to differentiate such progenitor cells from more mature cells with a lower proliferative capacity. CSFs therefore could be used therapeutically to encourage differentiation of malignant haemopoietic cells but there is concern that they might also promote leukaemia by enhancing proliferation of a malignant clone. This could be mediated by administration of exogenous factor, by enhanced expression of a factor or by an inappropriate cellular response to a factor.

Of the CSFs, G-CSF is the most effective in the induction of differentiation of murine leukaemic cells in vitro (Metcalf and Nicola, 1982). Human leukaemic cells have been shown to undergo terminal differentiation in vitro in response to rhG-CSF (Souza et al, 1986). Suppression of leukaemic stem cells has been achieved by the in vitro exposure of leukaemic cells to G-CSF. The cells so treated had reduced leukaemogenicity when subsequently transplanted into mice (Metcalf, 1984). In vitro myeloid leukaemia cells are dependent on exogenous CSF for continued growth (Metcalf, 1986). Autocrine secretion of GM-CSF has been demonstrated in vitro in a proportion of myeloid leukaemias and these endogenous factors were able to support leukaemic colonies from other cases of leukaemia (Young and Griffin, 1986). None of these cases had abnormalities of the long arm of chromosome 5, which has been shown to be the location of the GM-CSF gene.

A murine cell line has been described which is dependent on GM-CSF or IL-3 in vitro and which is not leukaemogenic in vivo. However when this line was transfected with a retrovirus coding for GM-CSF it became independent of exogenous factor, secreted GM-CSF and became leukaemogenic in mice (Lang et al, 1985). Feline M-CSF (CSF-1) receptor has strong sequence homology with the gene product of c-*fms* proto-oncogene (Scherr et al, 1985). In man, the c-*fms* locus has been assigned to the long arm of chromosome 5, deletion of which has been associated with a myelodysplastic syndrome frequently terminating in myeloid leukaemia (Wisniewski and Hirschhorn, 1983).

There are increased receptors for interleukin-2 on many adult T-cell leukaemias, hairy-cell leukaemias (Korsmeyer et al, 1983) and other non-T-cell leukaemias and lymphomas (Pui et al, 1987). Their significance in disease is not clear, as IL-2R have also been detected in serum from normal adults (Greene et al, 1986) although there may be a correlation between high levels and poor prognosis in some diseases (Pui et al, 1987).

In conclusion, it is important to develop an understanding of the relationship of the growth factors to normal and malignant haemopoiesis to allow their optimal and safe use. It also appears that, as they form a complex network, an appreciation of their inter-relationships and synergism with each other will almost certainly result in using growth factors in combination rather than as single agents. Although we can already see exciting potential for haemopoietic growth factors in the clinic, there is still much basic research to be done in defined systems in the laboratory to establish the subtle interplay of these factors in health and disease.

SUMMARY

Haemopoietic growth factors have for over two decades allowed experimentalists to grow haemopoietic bone marrow cells in vitro. With refinements in technique and the discovery of novel growth factors, all of the known haemopoietic lineages can now be grown in vitro. This has allowed a much greater understanding of the complex process of haemopoiesis from the haemopoietic stem cell to the mature, functioning end-cell.

The in vivo action of these growth factors has been harder to investigate. Although recombinant technology has afforded us the much greater quantities necessary for in vivo work, problems remain with administration because of effects on other tissues. Interpretation of results is difficult because of the complex inter-relationships which exist between factors. Some of these have been defined in vitro and it appears likely that they also operate in vivo.

Erythropoietin is a physiological regulator of erythropoiesis. It has been detected in vivo with levels responding appropriately to stress (i.e. elevated in anaemia) and, when administered in pharmacological doses, has been shown to correct anaemia. Granulocyte/macrophage colony-stimulating factor (GM-CSF) has been detected in vivo and may influence the production and function of granulocytes and macrophages, although how it is regulated is unknown. Granulocyte colony-stimulating factor (G-CSF) and macrophage colony-stimulating factor are more lineage-specific. Interleukin 3 (IL-3), although it has not been detected in vivo, may act on a primitive marrow precursor by expanding the population and making these cells more susceptible to other growth factors, such as GM-CSF. Interleukin 1 (IL-1) has been detected in vivo, does not appear to have any isolated action on bone marrow (except possibly radioprotection) but probably acts synergistically with other growth factors, such as G-CSF.

Interleukins 2, 4, 5 and 6 have not been detected in vivo. All have effects on B-cells. In addition IL-2 is an essential factor for the in vitro growth of T-cells and may have antitumour effects in vivo. IL-5 is an eosinophil growth factor in vitro. Megakaryocytopoiesis is also affected by humoral factors.

Factors, alone or in combination, may be useful to restore functional granulopoiesis when used therapeutically. Some can be used as anticancer agents, although there may be a risk of induction of haematological malignancy. Increased understanding of their physiological roles will allow a more rational use.

Acknowledgements

We would like to thank Dr Sue Watts for her help and advice in the preparation of this manuscript.

REFERENCES

Abbas AK (1987) Cellular interactions in the immune response. The roles of B lymphocytes and interleukin-4. *American Journal of Pathology* **129**: 26–33.

Anagnostou A, Barone J, Kedo A & Fried W (1977) Effect of erythropoietin therapy on the red cell volume of uraemic and non-uraemic rats. *British Journal of Haematology* **37**: 85–91.

Apperley JF, Jones L, Hale G et al (1986) Bone marrow transplantation for patients with chronic myeloid leukaemia: T-cell depletion with Campath-1 reduces the incidence of graft-versus-host disease but may increase the risk of leukaemic relapse. *Bone Marrow Transplantation* **1**: 53–66.

Balkwill FR (1985) Antitumour effects of interferons in animals. In Finter NB & Oldham RK (eds) *Interferon,4. In vivo and Clinical Studies*, pp 23–45. Amsterdam: Elsevier.

Balkwill FR & Smyth JF (1987) Interferons in cancer therapy: a reappraisal. *Lancet* **ii**: 317–319.

Balkwill FR, Griffin DB, Ward BG & Fiers W (1987) Human tumour xenografts treated with recombinant human tumour necrosis factor alone or in combination with interferons. *Cancer Research* **46**: 3990–3993.

Basten A & Beeson PB (1970) Mechanism of eosinophilia. II Role of the lymphocyte. *Journal of Experimental Medicine* **131**: 1288–1305.

Bell TV, Harley CB, Stetsko D & Sauder DN (1987) Expression of mRNA homologous to interleukin 1 in human epidermal cells. *Journal of Investigative Dermatology* **88**: 375–379.

Bendtzen K, Baek L, Berild D et al (1984) Demonstration of circulating leucocytic pyrogen/interleukin-1 during fever. *New England Journal of Medicine* **310**: 596.

Bergsagel DE, Hass RH & Messner HA (1986) Interferon α 2b in the treatment of chronic granulocytic leukaemia. *Seminars in Oncology* **13**: 29–35.

Bertoncello I, Bartelmez SH, Bradley TR et al (1986) Isolation and analysis of primitive hemopoietic progenitor cells on the basis of differential expression of Qa-m7 antigen. *Journal of Immunology* **136**: 3219–3224.

Beutler B & Cerami A (1986) Cachectin and tumour necrosis factor as two sides of the same biological coin. *Nature* **320**: 584–588.

Beutler B, Milsark IW & Cerami AC (1985) Passive immunisation against cachectin/tumour necrosis factor protects mice from lethal effects of endotoxins. *Science* **229**: 869–871.

Bino T, Edery H, Gertler A & Rosenberg H (1982) Involvement of the kidney in catabolism of human leucocyte interferon. *Journal of General Virology* **59**: 39–45.

Blick M, Sherwin SA, Rosenblum M & Gutterman (1987) Phase I study of recombinant tumor necrosis factor in cancer patients. *Cancer Research* **47**: 2986–2989.

Bonnard GD, Yasaka K & Jacobson D (1979) Ligand-activated T-cell growth factor induced proliferation: absorption of T-cell growth factor by activated T-cells. *Journal of Immunology* **125**: 2703–2708.

Bose S & Hickman J (1977) Role of carbohydrate moiety in determining the survival of interferon in the circulation. *Journal of Biological Chemistry* **252**: 8336–8337.

Bradley TR & Metcalf D (1966) The growth of mouse bone marrow cells in vitro. *Australian Journal of Experimental Biological Medical Science* **44**: 287–300.

Bradley TR, Metcalf D, Sumner MA & Stanley ER (1969) Characteristics of in vitro colony formation by cells from haemopoietic tissues. In Farnes P (ed.) *Hemic Cells In Vitro*, pp 22–35. Philadelphia: Williams & Wilkins.

Brouckaert PGG, Leroux-Roels GG, Guisez Y, Tavernier J & Fiers W (1986) In vivo anti-tumour activity of recombinant human and murine TNF, alone and in combination with murine IFN-γ, on a syngeneic murine melanoma. *International Journal of Cancer* **38**: 763–769.

Burgess AW (1985) Haematopoietic growth factors. In Ford RJ & Maizel AL (eds) *Mediators in Cell Growth and Differentiation*, pp 159–169. New York: Raven Press.

Campbell HD, Tucker WQJ, Hort Y et al (1987) Molecular cloning, nucleotide sequence, and expression of the gene encoding human eosinophil differentiation factor (interleukin 5). *Proceedings of the National Academy of Sciences USA* **84**: 6629–6633.

Carnot P & Deflandre C (1906) Sur l'activité hémapoiétique des différents organes au cours de la regénération du sang. *Comptes Rendus Hebdomadaires des Séances de l'Académie des Sciences* **143**: 432–436.

Clutterbuck EJ, Shields J, Gordon J et al (1987) Recombinant human interleukin 5 is an eosinophil differentiation factor but has no activity in standard human B cell growth factor assays. *European Journal of Immunology* **17**: 1743–1750.

Coffman R & Carty J (1986) A T cell activity that enhances polyclonal IgE production and its inhibition by interferon. *Journal of Immunology* **136**: 949–954.

Coutinho LH, Testa NG & Dexter TM (1986) The myelosuppressive effect of recombinant γ-interferon in short term and long term marrow cultures. *British Journal of Haematology* **63**: 517–524.

Das SK & Stanley ER (1982) Structure–function studies of a colony-stimulating factor (CSF-1). *Journal of Biological Chemistry* **257**: 13679–13684.

Dexter TM (1984) The message in the medium. *Nature* **309**: 746–747.

Dexter TM (1986) Growth factors: from the laboratory to the clinic. *Nature* **321**: 198.

Dexter TM & Moore M (1986) Growth and development in the haemopoietic system: the role of lymphokines and their possible therapeutic potential in disease and malignancy. *Carcinogenesis* **7**: 509–516.

Dexter TM, Garland J, Scott D, Scolnick E & Metcalf D (1980) Growth of factor dependent hemopoietic precursor cell lines. *Journal of Experimental Medicine* **152**: 1036–1047.

Dinarello CA (1986a) Studies on the biological properties of purified and recombinant human interleukin-1. *Methods and Findings in Experimental Clinical Pharmacology* **8**: 57–61.

Dinarello CA (1986b) Interleukin-1: amino acid sequences, multiple biological activities and comparison with tumor necrosis factor (cachetin). In Cruse JM & Lewis RE (eds) *The Year in Immunology*, pp 68–89. Basel: Karger.

Dinarello CA & Mier JW (1987) Lymphokines. *New England Journal of Medicine* **317**: 940–945.

Donahue RE, Wang EA, Stone DK et al (1986) Stimulation of haematopoiesis in primates by continuous infusion of recombinant human GM-CSF. *Nature* **321**: 872–875.

Erslev A (1953) Humoral regulation of red cell production. *Blood* **8**: 349–357.

Erslev A (1987) Erythropoietins coming of age. *New England Journal of Medicine* **316**: 101–103.

Eschbach JW, Egrie JC, Downing MR et al (1987) Correction of the anaemia of end-stage renal disease with recombinant human erythropoietin. *New England Journal of Medicine* **316**: 73–78.

Farrar WL, Johnson HM & Farrar JJ (1981) Regulation of the production of immune interferon and cytotoxic T lymphocytes by interleukin 2. *Journal of Immunology* **126**: 1120–1125.

Fleischmann J, Golde GW, Weisbart RH & Gasson JC (1986) Granulocyte-macrophage colony-stimulating factor enhances phagocytosis of bacteria by human neutrophils. *Blood* **68**: 708–711.

Gabrilove J, Jakubowski A, Grous J et al (1987) Initial results of a study of recombinant human granulocyte colony stimulating factor (rhuG-CSF) in cancer patients. *Experimental Hematology* **15**: 461.

Gahring L, Baltz M, Pepys MB & Daynes R (1984) Effect of ultraviolet irradiation on production of epidermal cell thymocyte-activating factor/interleukin 1 in vitro and in vivo. *Proceedings of the National Academy of Sciences USA* **81**: 1198–1202.

Gascon P, Zoumbos NC, Scala G et al (1985) Lymphokine abnormalities in aplastic anaemia: implications for the mechanism of action of antithymocyte globulin. *Blood* **65**: 407–413.

Gasson JC, Weisbart RH, Kaufman SE et al (1984) Purified human granulocyte-colony stimulating factor: direct action on neutrophils. *Science* **226:** 1339–1342.

Gery I, Gershon RK & Waksman BH (1972) Potentiation of the T-lymphocyte response to mitogens. 1. The responding cell. *Journal of Experimental Medicine* **136:** 128–142.

Goldwasser E, Ihle JN, Prystowsky MB & Van Zant G (1983) The effect of the interleukin-3 on haemopoietic precursor cells. In Golde DW & Marks PA (eds) *Normal and Neoplastic Haematopoiesis*, pp 301–309. New York: Liss.

Granelli-Piperno A, Andrus L & Reich E (1984) Antibodies to interleukin-2: effects on immune responses in vitro and in vivo. *Journal of Experimental Medicine* **160:** 738–750.

Greenberger JS, Sakakeeny MA, Humphries RK, Eaves CJ & Ecker RJ (1983) Demonstration of permanent factor dependent multipotential (erythroid/neutrophil/basophil) hemato-poietic progenitor cell lines. *Proceedings of the National Academy of Sciences USA* **80:** 2931–2935.

Greene WC, Leonard WJ, Depper JM, Nelson DL & Waldmann TR (1986) The human inter-leukin-2 receptor: normal and abnormal expression in T cells and in leukaemias induced by the human T-lymphotropic retroviruses. *Annals of Internal Medicine* **105:** 560–566.

Groopman JE, Mitsuyasu RT, DeLeo MJ et al (1987) Effect of recombinant human granulocyte-macrophage colony-stimulating factor on myelopoiesis in the acquired immunodeficiency syndrome. *New England Journal of Medicine* **317:** 593–599.

Gupta S (1986) Study of activated T cells in man. II. Interleukin 2 receptor and transferrin receptor expression on T cells and production of interleukin 2 in patients with acquired immune deficiency syndrome (AIDS) and AIDS-related complex. *Clinical Immunology and Immunopathology* **38:** 93–100.

Henney CS, Kuribayashi K, Kern DE & Gillis S (1981) Interleukin-2 augments natural killer cell activity. *Nature* **291:** 335–338.

Hernandez Bronchud M, Scargge JH, Thatcher N, Crowther D & Dexter TM (1987) Phase I/II study of recombinant human granulocyte colony-stimulating factor in patients receiving intensive chemotherapy for small cell lung cancer. *British Journal of Cancer* **56:** 809–814.

Hirano T, Taga T, Yasukawa K et al (1985) Human B-cell differentiation factor defined by an anti-peptide antibody and its possible role in autoantibody production. *Immunology* **84:** 228–231.

Hoffman R, Straneva J, Yang HH, Bruno E & Brandt J (1987) New insights into the regulation of human megakaryocytopoiesis. *Blood Cells* **13:** 75–86.

Hoffmann R, Mazur E, Bruno E & Floyd V (1981) Assay of an activity in the serum of patients with disorders of thrombopoiesis that stimulates formation of megakaryocyte colonies. *New England Journal of Medicine* **305:** 533–538.

Ihle JN (1986) Interleukin-3 regulation of the growth and differentiation of hemopoietic lymphoid stem cells. In Cruse JM & Lewis RE (eds) *The Year in Immunology*, pp 106–133. Basel: Karger.

Ihle JN, Keller J, Henderson L et al (1982) Procedures for the purification of interleukin 3 to homogeneity. *Journal of Immunology* **129:** 2431–2436.

Jubinsky PT & Stanley ER (1985) Purification of hemopoietin-1, a multilineage growth factor. *Proceedings of the National Academy of Sciences USA* **82:** 2764–2768.

Kaye WA, Adri MNS, Soeldner JS et al (1986) Acquired defect in interleukin-2 production in patients with type 1 diabetes mellitus. *New England Journal of Medicine* **315:** 920–924.

Kinashi T, Harada N, Severinson E et al (1986) Cloning of complementary DNA encoding T-cell replacing factor and identity with B-cell growth factor II. *Nature* **324:** 70–73.

Kindler V, Thorens B, de Kossodo S et al (1986) Stimulation of haematopoiesis in vivo by recombinant bacterial murine interleukin 3. *Proceedings of the National Academy of Sciences USA* **83:** 1001–1005.

Kluger MJ, Oppenheim JJ & Powanda MC (eds) (1985) *Progress in Leucocyte Biology, vol. 2. The Physiologic, Metabolic, and Immunologic Actions of Interleukin-1*. New York: Liss.

Korsmeyer SJ, Greene WC, Cossman J et al (1983) Rearrangement and expression of immuno-globulin genes and expression of Tac antigen in hairy cell leukaemia. *Proceedings of the National Academy of Sciences USA* **80:** 4522–4526.

Kupiec-Weglinski JW, Diamantstein T, Tilnet N & Strom TB (1986) Therapy with monoclonal antibody to interleukin 2 receptor spares suppressor T cells and prevents or reverses acute allograft rejection in rats. *Proceedings of the National Academy of Sciences USA* **83:** 2624–2627.

Lang RA, Metcalf D, Gough NM, Dunn AR & Gonda TJ (1985) Expression of a hemopoietic growth factor cDNA in a factor-dependent cell line results in autonomous growth and tumorigenicity. *Cell* **43:** 531–542.

Le PT, Tuck DT, Dinarello CA, Haynes BF & Singer KH (1987) Thymic epithelial cell-derived interleukin 1. *Journal of Immunology* (in press).

Liebson HJ, Geffer M, Zlotnik A, Marrack P & Kappler JW (1984) Role of interferon in antibody-producing responses. *Nature* **309:** 799–801.

Long MW, Williams N & McDonald TP (1982) Immature megakaryocytes in the mouse: in vitro relationships to megakaryocyte progenitor cells and mature megakaryocytes. *Journal of Cell Physiology* **112:** 339–344.

Lopez AF, Begley CG, Williamson DJ et al (1986) An eosinophil-specific colony-stimulating factor with activity for human cells. *Journal of Experimental Medicine* **163:** 1085–1099.

Lord BI, Molineux G, Testa NG et al (1986) The kinetic response of haemopoietic precursor cells, in vivo, to highly purified, recombinant interleukin-3. *Lymphokine Research* **5:** 97–104.

Lotze MT, Matory YL, Rayner AA et al (1986) Clinical effects and toxicity of interleukin-2 in patients with cancer. *Cancer* **58:** 2764–2772.

Lotzova E (1986) Therapeutic possibilities of virus-modified tumour cell extracts and interleukin-2 in human ovarian cancer. *Natural Immunity and Cell Growth Regulation* **5:** 277–282.

McDonald TP, Cottrell MB, Clift RE, Cullen WC & Lin FK (1987) High doses of recombinant erythropoietin stimulate platelet production in mice. *Experimental Hematology* **15:** 719–721.

Malkovsky M, Brenner MK, Hunt R et al (1987) T-cell depletion of allogeneic bone marrow prevents acceleration of graft-versus-host disease induced by exogenous interleukin 2. *Cellular Immunology* **103:** 476–480.

Marsh JC, Boggs DR, Cartwright GE & Wintrobe MM (1967) Neutrophil kinetics in acute infection. *Journal of Clinical Investigation* **46:** 1943–1953.

Masaoka T, Ohira M, Harada M et al (1986) Colony stimulating factor for bone marrow transplantation. *Experimental Hematology* **14:** 439.

Matsumoto M, Matsubara S, Matsuno T et al (1987) Protective effect on microbial infections in neutropenic mice. *Experimental Hematology* **15:** 558.

Mayer P, Lam C, Obenaus H, Liehl E & Besemer J (1987) Recombinant human GM-CSF induces leukocytosis and activates peripheral blood polymorphonuclear neutrophils in nonhuman primates. *Blood* **70:** 206–213.

Mazumber A & Rosenberg SA (1984) Successful immunotherapy of natural killer-resistant established pulmonary melanoma metastases by the intravenous adoptive transfer of syngeneic lymphocytes activated in vitro by interleukin 2. *Journal of Experimental Medicine* **159:** 495–507.

Metcalf D (1984) *The Hemopoietic Colony Stimulating Factors.* Amsterdam: Elsevier.

Metcalf D (1986) The molecular biology and functions of granulocyte-macrophage colony stimulating factors. *Blood* **67:** 257–267.

Metcalf D & Nicola NA (1982) Autoinduction of differentiation in WEHI-3B leukaemic cells. *International Journal of Cancer* **30:** 773–780.

Metcalf D & Stanley ER (1971) Haematological effects in mice of partially purified colony stimulating factor (CSF) prepared from human urine. *British Journal of Haematology* **21:** 481–492.

Metcalf D, Chan SH, Gunz SW, Vincent P & Ravich RBM (1971) Colony-stimulating factor and inhibitor levels in acute granulocytic leukaemia. *Blood* **43:** 847–859.

Metcalf D, Begley CG, Williamson DJ et al (1987a) Hemopoietic responses in mice injected with purified recombinant murine GM-CSF. *Experimental Hematology* **15:** 1–10.

Metcalf D, Begley CG, Nicola NA & Johnson GR (1987b) Quantitative responsiveness of murine haemopoietic populations in vitro and in vivo to recombinant multi-CSF (IL3). *Experimental Hematology* **15:** 288–295.

Miyake T, Kung CK-H & Goldwasser E (1977) Purification of human erythropoietin. *Journal of Biological Chemistry* **252:** 5558–5564.

Mizutani S, Watt SM, Robertson D et al (1987) Cloning of human subcapsular cortex epithelial cells with T-lymphocyte binding sites and haemopoietic growth factor activity. *Proceedings of the National Academy of Sciences USA* **84:** 4999–5003.

Mochizuki DY, Eisenman JR, Conlon PJ, Larsen AD & Tushinski RJ (1987) Interleukin 1 regulates hematopoietic activity, a role previously ascribed to hemapoietin 1. *Proceedings of the National Academy of Sciences USA* **84**: 5267–5271.

Moore MAS & Warren DJ (1987) Synergy of interleukin 1 and granulocyte colony-stimulating factor: in vivo stimulation of stem cell recovery and hematopoietic regeneration following 5-fluorouracil treatment of mice. *Proceedings of the National Academy of Sciences USA* **84**: 7134–7139.

Motoyshi K, Takaku F, Maekawa T et al (1986) Protective effect of partially purified human urinary colony-stimulating factor on granulocytopenia after antitumor chemotherapy. *Experimental Hematology* **14**: 1069–1075.

Munker R, Gasson J, Ogawa M & Koeffler HP (1986) Recombinant human TNF induces production of granulocyte-macrophage colony-stimulating factor. *Nature* **323**: 79–82.

Murray HW, Rubin BY & Rothermal CD (1983) Killing of intracellular *Leishmania donovani* by lymphokine-stimulated human mononuclear phagocytes: evidence that interferon-γ is the activating lymphokine. *Journal of Clinical Investigation* **72**: 1506–1510.

Myers AM & Robinson WA (1975) Colony stimulating factor levels in human serum and urine following chemotherapy. *Proceedings of the Society for Experimental Biology and Medicine* **3**: 694–700.

Neff MS, Goldberg J, Slifkin RF et al (1981) A comparison of androgens in patients on hemodialysis. *New England Journal of Medicine* **304**: 871–875.

Neta R, Douches S & Oppenheim JJ (1986) Interleukin 1 is a radioprotector. *Journal of Immunology* **136**: 2483–2485.

Neta R, Douches S & Oppenheim JJ (1987) In vivo effects and interactions of rTNF-α and rIL 1β in radioprotection, induction of CSF and fibrinogen. *Immunobiology* **175**: 23.

Neufeld EF & Ashwell G (1980) Carbohydrate recognition systems for receptor-mediated pinocytosis. In Lennart W (ed.) *The Biochemistry of Glycoproteins and Proteoglycans*, p 241. New York: Plenum.

Nienhuis AW, Donahue RE, Karlsson S et al (1987) Recombinant human granulocyte-macrophage colony-stimulating factor (GM-CSF) shortens the period of neutropenia after autologous bone marrow transplantation in a primate model. *Journal of Clinical Investigation* **80**: 573–577.

Noma Y, Sideras P, Naito T et al (1986) Cloning of cDNA encoding the murine IgG1 induction factor by a novel strategy using SP6 promoter. *Nature* **319**: 640–646.

Okabe T, Sato N, Kondo Y et al (1978) Establishment and characterisation of a human cancer cell line that produces human colony-stimulating factor. *Cancer Research* **38**: 3910–3917.

Oppenheim JJ, Kovacs EJ, Matsushima K & Durum SK (1986) There is more than one interleukin 1. *Immunology Today* **7**: 45–56.

Pace JL, Russell SW, Torres BA et al (1983) Recombinant mouse γ interferon induces the priming step in macrophage activation for tumor cell killing. *Journal of Immunology* **130**: 2011–2013.

Pfizenmaier K, Scheurich P, Daubener W et al (1984) Quantitative representation of all T cells committed to develop into cytotoxic effector cells and for interleukin-2 activity-producing helper cells within murine T lymphocyte subsets. *European Journal of Immunology* **14**: 33–39.

Piguet PF, Grau G, Allet B & Vassali P (1987) Tumour necrosis factor (TNF) is an important mediator of the mortality and morbidity induced by the graft-versus-host reaction (GVHR). *Immunobiology* **175**: 27.

Pluznik DH & Sachs L (1965) The cloning of normal 'mast' cells in tissue culture. *Journal of Cellular and Comparative Physiology* **66**: 319–324.

Pui C-H, Ip SH, Kung P, Dodge RK & Berard CW (1987) High serum interleukin-2 receptor levels are related to advanced disease and a poor outcome in childhood non-Hodgkin's lymphoma. *Blood* **70**: 624–628.

Quesada JR, Reuben J, Manning JT et al (1984) Alpha interferon for induction of remission in hairy-cell leukaemia. *New England Journal of Medicine* **310**: 15–18.

Quesenberry PJ (1986) Synergistic hematopoietic growth factors. *International Journal of Cellular Cloning* **4**: 3–15.

Quesenberry PJ, Ihle JN & McGrath E (1985) The effect of interleukin-3 and GM-CSA-2 on megakaryocyte and myeloid clonal colony formation. *Blood* **65**: 214–217.

Reissman KR (1950) Studies on the mechanisms of erythropoietic stimulation in parabiotic rats during hypoxia. *Blood* **5**: 373–380.

Robb RJ & Smith KA (1981) Human T-cell growth factor is glycosylated. *Molecular Immunology* **18**: 1087–1094.

Robinson WA, Metcalf D & Bradley TR (1967) Stimulation by normal and leukemic mouse sera of colony formation in vitro by mouse bone marrow cells. *Journal of Cellular Physiology* **69**: 83–92.

Rosenberg SA, Mule JJ, Speiss PJ, Reichert CM & Schwarz SL (1985) Regression of established pulmonary metastases and subcutaneous tumour mediated by the systemic administration of high-dose recombinant interleukin-2. *Journal of Experimental Medicine* **161**: 1169–1188.

Rosenberg SA, Spiess P & Lafreniere R (1986) A new approach to the adoptive immunotherapy of cancer with tumour-infiltrating lymphocytes. *Science* **233**: 1318–1321.

Rosenberg SA, Lotze MT, Muul LM et al (1987) A progress report on the treatment of 157 patients with advanced cancer using lymphokine activated killer cells and interleukin-2 or high-dose interleukin-2 alone. *New England Journal of Medicine* **316**: 889–897.

Ruggiero V & Baglioni C (1987) Synergistic anti-proliferative activity of interleukin 1 and tumor necrosis factor. *Journal of Immunology* **138**: 661–663.

Sanderson CJ, Warren DJ & Strath M (1985) Identification of a lymphokine that stimulates eosinophil differentiation in vitro. Its relation to interleukin 3, and functional properties of eosinophils produced in cultures. *Journal of Experimental Medicine* **162**: 60–74.

Scala G, Kuang YD, Hall RE, Muhmore AV & Oppenheim JJ (1984) Accessory cell function of human B cells. Production of both interleukin-1-like activity and an interleukin-1 inhibitory factor by an EBV-transformed human B cell line. *Journal of Experimental Medicine* **159**: 1637–1652.

Scherr CJ, Rettenmier CW, Sacca R et al (1985) The c-*fms* proto-oncogene product is related to the receptor for the mononuclear phagocyte growth factor, CSF-1. *Cell* **41**: 665–676.

Selby P, Hobbs S, Fearon K et al (1988) Tumour necrosis factor in man: clinical and biological observations. *British Journal of Cancer* **56**: 803–809.

Shadduck RK & Waheed A (1986) Access of CSF-1 to hemopoietic progenitor cells in vivo. *Blood* **68**: 179a.

Shadduck RK, Carsten AL, Chikkappa A et al (1986) Regulation of diffusion-chamber granulopoiesis by colony-stimulating factor. *Experimental Hematology* **14**: 812–818.

Shadduck RK, Waheed A, Boegel F et al (1987) The effect of colony stimulating factor-1 in vivo. *Blood Cells* **13**: 49–63.

Shimamura M, Kobayashi Y, Yuo A et al (1987) Effect of human recombinant granulocyte colony-stimulating factor on hematopoietic injury in mice induced by 5-fluorouracil. *Blood* **69**: 353–355.

Smith CA & Rennick DM (1986) Characterisation of a murine lymphokine distinct from interleukin 2 and interleukin 3 (IL-3) possessing a T-cell growth factor activity and a mast-cell growth factor activity that synergises with IL-3. *Proceedings of the National Academy of Sciences* **83**: 1857–1861.

Sonoda Y et al (1988) Analysis in serum-free culture of the targets of recombinant human haemopoietic growth factors: Interleukin 3 and granulocyte/macrophage-colony-stimulating factor are specific for early developmental stages. *Proceedings of the National Academy of Science of the USA* **85**: 4360–4364.

Souza LM, Boone TC, Gabrilove J et al (1986) Recombinant human granulocyte colony-stimulating factor: effects on normal and leukaemic myeloid cells. *Science* **232**: 61–65.

Spivak JL, Smith RRL & Ihle JN (1985) Interleukin-3 promotes the in vitro proliferation of murine pluripotent haematopoietic stem cells. *Journal of Cellular Physiology* **76**: 1613.

Stanley ER, Bartocci A, Patinkin D, Rosendaal M & Bradley TR (1986) Regulation of very primitive, multipotent hemopoietic cells by hemopoietin-1. *Cell* **45**: 667–674.

Stone-Wolff DS, Yip YK, Kelker KC et al (1984) Interrelationships of human interferon-gamma with lymphotoxin and monocyte cytotoxin. *Journal of Experimental Medicine* **159**: 828–843.

Straneva JE, Yang HH, Bruno E & Hoffman R (1986) Separate factors control cytoplasmic maturation of human megakaryocytes. In Liams N, Levin J & Evatt BL (eds) *Megakaryocyte Development and Function*, pp 253–258. New York: Alan R Liss.

Straneva JE, Yang HH, Hui SL, Bruno E & Hoffman R (1987) Effects of megakaryocyte colony-stimulating factor on terminal cytoplasmic maturation of human megakaryocytes. *Experimental Hematology* **15**: 657–663.

Surgenor DM (1987) The patient's blood is the safest blood. *New England Journal of Medicine* **316**: 542–544.

Takatsu K, Kikuchi Y, Takahashi T et al (1987) Interleukin 5, a T-cell-derived B-cell differentiation factor also induces cytotoxic T lymphocytes. *Proceedings of the National Academy of Sciences USA* **84**: 4234–4238.

Takeda K, Iwamoto S, Sugimoto H et al (1986) Identity of differentiation factor and tumour necrosis factor. *Nature* **323**: 338–340.

Tamura M, Hattori K, Nomura H et al (1987) Induction of neutrophilic granulocytosis in mice by administration of purified human native granulocyte colony-stimulating factor (G-CSF). *Biochemical and Biophysical Research Communications* **142**: 454–460.

Van Damme J, Van Beemen J, Decock B et al (1987a) Identification of the 26-kD protein, interferon 2 (IFN 2), as a B cell hybridoma/plasmacytoma growth factor induced by interleukin 1 and tumor necrosis factor. *Journal of Experimental Medicine* **165**: 914–919.

Van Damme J, Caybhas S, Than Snick J et al (1987b) Purification and characterization of human fibroblast-derived hybridoma growth factor identical to T-cell-derived B-cell stimulatory factor-2 (Interleukin-6). *European Journal of Biochemistry* **168**: 543–550.

Vogel SN, Douches SD, Kaufman EN & Neta R (1987) Induction of colony stimulating factor in vivo by recombinant interleukin-1 and recombinant tumour necrosis factor. *Journal of Immunology* **138**: 2143–2146.

Welte K, Bonilla MA, Gillio AP et al (1987a) Recombinant human granulocyte colony stimulating factor. Effects on hematopoiesis in normal and cyclophosphamide-treated primates. *Journal of Experimental Medicine* **165**: 941–948.

Welte K, Bonilla MA, Gillio A et al (1987b) In vivo effects of recombinant human G-CSF in therapy induced neutropenias in primates. *Experimental Hematology* **15**: 460.

West WH, Tauer KW, Yanelli JR et al (1987) Constant-infusion recombinant interleukin-2 in adoptive immunotherapy of advanced cancer. *New England Journal of Medicine* **316**: 898–906.

Williams N, Jackson H, Iscove NN & Dukes PP (1984) The role of erythropoietin, thrombopoietic stimulating factor, and myeloid colony-stimulating factors on murine megakaryocyte colony formation. *Experimental Hematology* **12**: 734–740.

Winearls CG, Oliver DO, Pippard MJ et al (1986) Effect of human erythropoietin derived from recombinant DNA on the anaemia of patients maintained by chronic haemodialysis. *Lancet* **ii**: 1175–1178.

Wisniewski LP & Hirschhorn K (1983) Acquired partial deletions of the long arm of chromosome 5 in hematologic disorders. *American Journal of Hematology* **15**: 295–310.

Wong GG, Witek JS, Temple PA et al (1985) Human GM-CSF: molecular cloning of the complementary DNA and purification of the natural and recombinant proteins. *Science* **228**: 810–815.

Yang HH, Bruno E & Hoffman R (1986) Studies of human megakaryocytopoiesis using an anti-megakaryocyte colony-stimulating factor antiserum. *Journal of Clinical Investigation* **77**: 1873–1880.

Yang YC, Donahue R, Ogawa M et al (1987) Biological properties of human interleukin-3. *Abstracts of Stem Cells and Autologous Bone Marrow Transplantation, Vancouver, 1987.*

Yokota T, Otsuki T, Mosmann T et al (1986) Isolation and characterisation of a human interleukin cDNA clone, homologous to mouse B-cell stimulatory factor 1, that expresses B-cell- and T-cell-stimulating activities. *Proceedings of the National Academy of Sciences USA* **83**: 5894–5898.

Young DC & Griffin JD (1986) Autocrine secretion of GM-CSF in acute myeloblastic leukaemia. *Blood* **68**: 1178–1181.

Young NS, Leonard E & Platanias L (1987) Lymphocytes and lymphokines in aplastic anaemia: pathogenic role and implications for pathogenesis. *Blood Cells* **13**: 87–100.

Yron I, Wood TA, Spiess P & Rosenberg SA (1980) In vitro growth of murine T cells: the isolation and growth of lymphoid cells infiltrating syngeneic solid tumors. *Journal of Immunology* **125**: 238–245.

Zlotnik A, Fischer M, Roehm N & Zipori D (1987a) Evidence for effects of interleukin 4 (B cell stimulatory factor 1) on macrophages: enhancement of antigen presenting ability of bone marrow-derived macrophages. *Journal of Immunology* **138**: 4275–4279.

Zlotnik A, Ransom J, Frank G, Fischer M & Howard M (1987b) Interleukin 4 is a growth factor for activated thymocytes: possible role in T-cell ontogeny. *Proceedings of the National Academy of Sciences USA* **84:** 3856–3860.

Zoumbos N, Gascon P, Djeu J & Young N (1985) Interferon is a mediator of hematopoietic suppression in aplastic anaemia in vitro and possibly in vivo. *Proceedings of the National Academy of Sciences USA* **82:** 188–192.

7

Paroxysmal nocturnal haemoglobinuria

BRUNO ROTOLI
LUCIO LUZZATTO

Paroxysmal nocturnal haemoglobinuria (PNH) is an intriguing haematological disorder first identified by Strübing in 1882 and later described in
greater detail by Marchiafava and Nazari in 1911 and Micheli in 1931. Its
prevalence is estimated at about one case in 500 000 persons (Crosby, 1953).
By 1973 more than 500 cases were collected from the literature (Polli et al,
1973); however this figure must be a vast underestimate, since there is no
reason today for publishing single cases or even further series of patients.
    Although the disease affects several cell lineages the most prominent
clinical manifestation is intravascular haemolysis due to an intrinsic red cell
defect. Therefore, PNH has been traditionally classified as a haemolytic
disorder. When it was realized that white cells and platelets were also
involved, inclusion among myeloproliferative or myelodysplastic syndromes was proposed (Dameshek, 1969). However, the frequent finding
of moderate to severe pancytopenia, the reduced number of white cells and
platelets without evidence of accelerated peripheral destruction, and the
results of in vitro cultures all point to a close relationship with acquired
aplastic anaemia, thus justifying the inclusion of PNH in this volume. The
problem of how PNH relates to acquired aplastic anaemia is not merely
academic, since a correct nosology may help in deciding on the most appropriate treatment.
    In this chapter, clinical and haematological aspects of PNH will be briefly
summarized, since little needs to be added to previous comprehensive
reviews of this topic (Dacie and Lewis, 1972; Sirchia and Lewis, 1975; Rosse
and Parker, 1985). More attention will be paid to the identification of a
number of cell surface molecules capable of protecting cells from complement lysis and which may be altered in PNH, and to the results of in vitro
culture studies, since in the last few years these have provided some insight
into the basis and mechanism of haemolysis. We also present a speculative
model of the possible relationship of PNH to acquired aplastic anaemia and
to myeloproliferative disorders. Finally, we shall briefly review the
therapeutic approaches to PNH, including bone marrow transplantation.

CLINICAL ASPECTS

Presentation

The most common presentation of PNH, observed in about 50% of patients, is that of a young adult with several months' history of weakness and pallor, occasionally passing dark urine in the morning, who is found to be mildly jaundiced, moderately anaemic, with a reduced number of white blood cells and platelets, and a reticulocytosis which is never very marked. However, none of these findings is uniformly present. Rare cases of PNH in childhood (Resegotti and Givone, 1962) and some cases in patients over 50 years old have been observed; jaundice may be transient or absent; anaemia may sometimes be much more severe and the reticulocyte count may be low in hypoplastic forms; white blood cells and platelets may be normal for some time, before they decrease in numbers.

Although dark urine may occur never or just once, this sign, when present, is a real clue to the diagnosis. Typically, port-wine or cola-coloured urine is passed in the morning, while later during the day the urine becomes clear. Since colour is not light red but dark and clots are never present, confusion with haematuria is unlikely. However, doctors who have not seen the urine may think not of a blood disease, but rather of a liver disease. Additional features of PNH are unexplained recurrent abdominal pain, venous thrombosis, and increased susceptibility to infections.

Of the 50% of patients who do not show the typical presentation, a substantial proportion present with pancytopenia and consequent complications in the way of bleeding and infections, mimicking a severe hypoplastic or frank aplastic anaemia. In these cases jaundice, reticulocytosis and dark urine are absent but a few signs may be clues to the current diagnosis. First of all, although there may be no signs of excessive haemolysis, there are signs of active erythropoiesis which would be unexpected in typical acquired aplastic anaemia: for instance, mild reticulocytosis, polychromasia in blood smears, persistence of erythroid tissue in bone marrow, and lack of the serum bilirubin level reduction usually observed in aplastic patients. Secondly, serum haptoglobin is low and lactic dehydrogenase may be raised. Finally, although a mild enlargement of the spleen is present in less than 50% of patients with PNH, its presence in aplastic patients deserves further investigation.

In most patients with PNH the average interval between onset of symptoms and diagnosis is 1–2 years. Since simple, sensitive and specific diagnostic tests are available, the reason for the delayed diagnosis is somewhat curious and it must be attributed to the fact that doctors often do not think of this disease when assessing anaemic patients. Indeed, when PNH is suspected, laboratory confirmation is simple: it is sufficient, for clinical purposes, to carry out the Ham test with the appropriate controls (see below), and to stain the urinary sediment for haemosiderin.

Course

The clinical course of PNH results from the variable expression of four basic components of its pathophysiology: hyperhaemolysis, bone marrow failure, infection and thrombosis.

Hyperhaemolysis

PNH is characterized by chronic haemolysis with sudden exacerbations. The shortened red cell survival is usually not adequately compensated for, resulting in overt anaemia. Pallor and jaundice fluctuate; since the disorder is chronic, patients usually tolerate the anaemia rather well, except during exacerbations, when fatigue and dyspnoea set in.

Exacerbations, heralded by haemoglobinuria, are often apparently spontaneous; thus far, there is no good explanation for the trigger effect of sleep. A number of other trigger factors have been identified. Probably all of these factors cause hyperhaemolysis by activating molecules capable of determining red cell destruction, i.e. the complement system. This may happen directly, as in the case of infection, strenuous exercise or stress, or indirectly, for instance after blood transfusion. Since donor red cells survive normally in PNH patients, there must be ways whereby autologous red cell destruction is activated. One possible mechanism is complement activation by immune reactions against white cell or platelet antigens in multiply transfused patients. In this case haemolysis occurs during or immediately after transfusion, and it is associated with some degree of clinical reaction. Another possible explanation is the presence of activated complement in the plasma of stored blood. Third, since some patients experience morning haemoglobinuria soon after a course of intensive transfusions even if washed or filtered red cells were used and there was no clinical reaction, it is possible that the increased autologous red cell lysis is mediated by modifications of physical properties of the plasma resulting from the restoration of higher haematocrit (see below).

Another cause of exacerbation is iron treatment. Because of permanent haemosiderinuria PNH patients may develop iron deficiency which makes the anaemic state worse. Effective iron replacement may be followed by increased red cell lysis. There are at least two explanations for this phenomenon: firstly, a cohort of young cells includes a larger proportion of PNH cells (Rosse and Gutterman, 1970) and secondly, the increased haematocrit acts as a mechanism of sensitization for PNH cells to be destroyed.

Bone marrow failure

Insufficient bone marrow haemopoietic function is inferred in PNH patients from granulocytopenia and thrombocytopenia with normal in vivo cell survival, and from a discrepancy between the rate of haemolysis and the extent of compensation through increased red cell production. It is also documented by in vitro culture studies (see below). It is customary to classify patients with PNH as having either a haemolytic form, in which the signs of red cell destruction dominate the clinical picture, or as having an aplastic form in which pancytopenia and its consequences are the main findings (although all sorts of intermediate forms are possible). Conversely, it is good practice to do a Ham test on the blood of any patient with hypoplastic or aplastic anaemia. For unknown reasons, PNH patients may show complete or partial *selective* bone marrow aplasia; the authors have seen PNH patients with agranulocytosis and normal platelet count, or with amegakaryocytic thrombocytopenia and normal white blood cells. The clinical picture of PNH patients with the aplastic form is dominated by transfusion dependence, haemorrhage and infections.

Infections

Increased sensitivity to bacterial infections is variably seen in PNH patients. Obviously, it depends on the number of circulating neutrophils, thus it is more severe in the aplastic form. Besides reduced numbers, functional abnormalities of white cells have been observed in PNH patients, with reduced neutrophil alkaline phosphatase activity, defective migration, decreased sticking to filters, defective phagocytosis, increased lysis in acidified serum or by antibodies (Lewis and Dacie, 1965; Penny and Galton, 1966; Aster and Enright, 1969; Craddock et al, 1976; Brubaker et al, 1977). These qualitative changes may contribute to the incidence and the severity of infectious episodes. In a patient with PNH with a two-lineage hypoplasia (severe transfusion-dependent anaemia and neutropenia, with normal platelet count), a number of severe skin infections, and a colonic ulcer requiring partial right colectomy, occurred within a few years (authors' personal observation). In addition to quantitative and qualitative abnormalities of neutrophils, reticuloendothelial blockade through chronic haemolysis may also contribute to impaired resistance against certain infectious agents.

Venous thrombosis

The frequent occurrence of venous thrombosis in PNH patients has been attributed to enhanced platelet activity, which in turn may result from both intrinsic and extrinsic causes. In PNH patients platelets carry the same membrane abnormality as red cells, i.e. they are abnormally sensitive to activated complement fractions, which produce platelet aggregation. Adenosine diphosphate released into the circulation by disrupted red cells may be responsible for intravascular platelet activation. Red cell ghosts may cause small vessel occlusion by themselves. The most severe and not unusual form of thrombosis in PNH is progressive diffuse hepatic vein thrombosis (Budd–Chiari syndrome), which is often rapidly fatal. As a rough rule, patients with the haemolytic form and a normal platelet count are likely to develop venous thrombosis, whereas patients with the aplastic form more often develop infectious complications.

Association with other haematological disorders

PNH has been reported in association with hypoplastic or aplastic anaemia, myeloproliferative syndromes and acute leukaemias. Considering the relative rarity of these conditions and of PNH, such associations can hardly be regarded as fortuitous.

Aplastic anaemia

As already mentioned at the beginning of this chapter, a substantial number of typical cases of PNH show, at diagnosis, unequivocal signs of bone marrow failure (Lewis and Dacie, 1967). In addition, there are sequential associations between PNH and acquired aplastic anaemia. PNH patients may develop acquired aplastic anaemia during the course of their disease and perhaps lose their PNH abnormality or, in the opposite direction, acquired aplastic anaemia patients may acquire the PNH abnormality and sometimes experience an amelioration of their anaemic state (Sicigliano et al, 1987). Finally, there is epidemiological evidence of increased prevalance of PNH in areas where acquired aplastic anaemia is frequent, e.g. in Thailand (Kruatrachue et al, 1978). Thus, connections between PNH and acquired aplastic anaemia are strong enough to prompt a search for a pathogenetic link (see below).

Myeloproliferative syndromes

A number of cases of myeloproliferative (MPD) or myelodysplastic (MDS) syndromes with positive Ham test and signs of intravascular haemolysis have also been reported. We have previously reviewed 29 such cases, including

Table 1. Association of PNH with myeloproliferative disorders.

Condition	Number of collected cases
Acute myeloid leukaemia	15
Erythroleukaemia	6
Chronic myeloid leukaemia	8
Idiopathic myelofibrosis	7
Megakaryocytic myelosis	1
Polycythaemia vera	Not reported

For references, see Luzzatto et al (1979) and text.

personal observations (Luzzatto et al, 1979) and additional patients were found in the recent literature (Table 1). We found a positive Ham test in 11 out of 113 patients with MPD studied in Ibadan (Nigeria) and Naples (Italy), lysis in acidified serum ranging from 2 to 12%. However, the patient population was not totally unselected, since it included the two index cases of erythremic myelosis (AML-M6) that prompted the study. It is hard to assess the clinical significance of the PNH defect during the course of these diseases; in most patients signs of intravascular haemolysis were not detectable. But, as with acquired aplastic anaemia, the connection between PNH and MDS is intriguing and could be a clue for a better understanding of the reasons for which the PNH abnormality may become apparent.

Acute leukaemia

The occurrence of acute leukaemia in patients with typical PNH has been observed (Holden and Lichtman, 1969; Carmel et al, 1970; Cowall et al,

1979; Hirsch et al, 1981; Katahira et al, 1983; Krause, 1983; Devine et al, 1987). Although this is a rare event (probably the proportion of PNH patients developing acute leukaemia is similar to that of patients with acquired aplastic anaemia), it is enough to make us consider PNH as a preleukaemic state.

Outcome

In the majority of patients the PNH lesion is permanent, and even the subtype of PNH (haemolytic or aplastic) does not change. In a minority of patients the lesion is transient. Occasional cases of spontaneous recovery were reported in the past (Dacie and Lewis, 1972); in addition, the development of aplastic anaemia or acute leukemia may be associated with loss of the PNH abnormality. Finally, a few patients with PNH who have undergone allogeneic or syngeneic bone marrow transplantation have experienced complete haematological remission associated with disappearance of the PNH abnormality.

HAEMATOLOGY

Ham test

Following the fundamental studies of Ham (Ham and Dingle, 1939), Rosse and Dacie (1966), it was clearly demonstrated that PNH red cells (and other blood cells) are abnormally sensitive to activated complement. This is the basis of several diagnostic procedures called the sugar/water test, the sucrose test, the Ham test, the antibody-mediated complement lysis test and the thrombin test. In fact, these methods only differ as to the pathway used to activate complement. In most people's opinion, including ours, the acidified serum lysis test (Ham), appropriately carried out, remains the gold standard.

Although technical aspects of these tests will not be discussed here, (for which the reader is referred to laboratory handbooks), the need for appropriate controls in the Ham test must be emphasized. In PNH haemolysis occurs with the patient's red cells, but not with normal red cells, both in the patient's own and in donor (compatible) sera, provided that serum is fresh, acidified and not heated (Table 2). Haemolysis of normal (compatible red cells in patient's acidified serum is evidence for acid haemolysins (as is sometimes found in autoimmune haemolytic anaemia). In PNH, haemolysis is *not* associated with agglutination, which again would indicate presence of anti-erythrocyte antibodies.

A rare form of congenital dyserythropoietic anaemia (type II or hereditary erythroblastic multinuclearity with positive acid serum test; HEMPAS) is also associated with a positive Ham test (Rosse et al, 1974). However, in HEMPAS the patient's own serum is ineffective; only a proportion of normal sera shows lytic activity following acidification; and, when present, lysis in normal acidified serum is associated with agglutination.

Table 2. The value and pitfalls of the Ham test.

Red blood cells from patients with:	PNH	CDA-II	AIHA
Normal untreated serum	trace	–	–
Normal acidified serum	++	++*	–
Patient's acidified serum	+	–	++
Heated acidified serum	–	–	–
Concomitant agglutination	–	+	+

PNH = paroxysmal nocturnal haemoglobinuria; CDA-II = congenital dyserythropoietic anaemia type II AIHA = autoimmune haemolytic anaemia with acid haemolysins.
* Only with a portion of sera from normal compatible subjects.

Although setting up negative controls for the Ham test is easy, a positive control requires cells from a known PNH patient. Artificial modifications of the red cell membrane (2-amino-ethylisothiouronium bromide treated red cells) can mimic the PNH lesion (Sirchia et al, 1964), but the procedure is delicate and time-consuming. For practical purposes, it is sufficient to be sure that the sera are fresh and that the pH after acidification is in the correct range (6.7–7).

The sensitivity of the Ham test is high; as little as 2% haemolysis can be detected and is sufficient for diagnosis. The authors recommend measuring the haemolysis quantitatively. There is no direct correlation between percentage of haemolysis and severity of anaemia. In part this may result from the rapid disapparance from the circulation of a large number of abnormal cells. When anaemia is pronounced and the Ham test only weakly positive, it must be inferred that anaemia is mainly aregenerative, as seen in the aplastic form of PNH.

Red cell survival

The ^{51}Cr half-life is usually shortened in PNH patients, although not markedly. Since this method is based on random labelling of mature red cells with ^{51}Cr, it probably underestimates haemolysis because PNH cells have in part already disappeared from the circulation. Because of chronic, predominantly intravascular haemolysis, loss of ^{51}Cr with urine is usually apparent. However, some extravascular haemolysis also occurs. In multiply transfused patients the spleen may be enlarged and the finding of a splenic uptake of labelled red cells may be regarded as an indication for splenectomy (Figure 1).

Haemosiderinuria

As in other chronic intravascular haemolytic disorders (e.g. cold agglutinin disease), even in the absence of detectable haemoglobinuria, haemosiderinuria is constantly present and may cause iron deficiency. Iron deficiency is more frequent in haemolytic PNH; in the aplastic form the urinary loss is

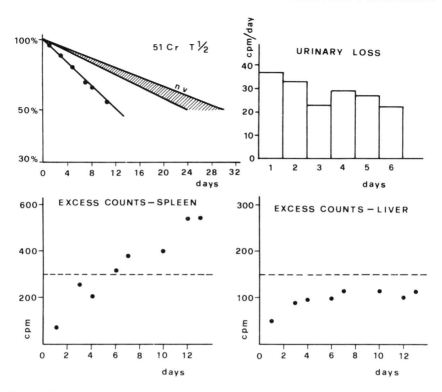

Figure 1. Decreased red cell life span in a multiply transfused PNH patient with splenomegaly. **Top left:** ^{51}Cr-labelled red cell survival study; **top right:** ^{51}Cr in urine, indicating intravascular haemolysis; **bottom:** time course of radioactivity in spleen and liver, showing evidence of coexistent extravascular (splenic) haemolysis.

usually insufficient to balance the transfusional intake, and therapeutic iron chelation may be needed.

PATHOGENESIS

Evidence for a specific subset of abnormal blood cells in PNH patients

Consideration of the haematological findings has for some time led to the notion that more than one red cell population exists in the peripheral blood of PNH patients. Several pieces of circumstantial evidence can be quoted. First of all, the cells lysed in the Ham test (or in similar diagnostic tests) are a finite fraction of the total, that is, red cells that have escaped lysis cannot be lysed if tested again, suggesting the coexistence of two types of red cells, some sensitive and some not sensitive to acid serum lysis. Secondly, ^{51}Cr red cell survival studies may show a two-slope profile of red cell disapparance, suggesting two populations with different survival times (Lewis et al, 1960) but this evidence is not conclusive. It is conceivable that in both the Ham test and ^{51}Cr survival studies a threshold effect gives the impression of two or even more populations when only one exists.

Rosse and Dacie (1966) demonstrated that PNH red cell lysis by antibody-activated complement was linear with the amount of complement. Since most patients showed two slopes separated by a plateau, this was considered as evidence that more than one red cell population is present in PNH. The analysis of the rather complex curves seen in some patients gave rise to the hypothesis that some PNH patients may have several cell populations, one normal (PNH-0) or almost normal (PNH-I), a second one three- to five-fold more sensitive to complement (PNH-II), and a third one 15- to 25-fold more sensitive to complement (PNH-III), possibly composed of two subpopulations, IIIa and IIIb (Chow et al, 1986). In the majority of cases only two populations are present (PNH-I and PNH-II or PNH-I and PNH-III). The possibility that the differences seen in this test could be secondarily acquired or in some way induced by the experimental conditions employed cannot be ruled out.

A formal proof of the existence of two distinct populations of red cells was obtained in 1970 when, in two female patients with PNH who were also heterozygous for two different glucose-6-phosphate dehydrogenase (G6PD) variants, only one type of enzyme was found in the supernatant after acidified serum lysis, while both types were present in whole blood (Oni et al, 1970). This study confirmed the presence of more than one population of red cells in PNH, and it proved the monoclonal origin of the population with the PNH defect. Subsequently, in vitro culture studies made it possible to test the two-population model in another direct way. The model predicts that erythroid cell progenitors (BFU-E) must also be of two kinds, normal and PNH. Each erythroid burst would then have to consist entirely of either normal or PNH cells. Using two independent criteria Rotoli et al (1984) showed that two kinds of burst can be grown from PNH patients, one normal and the other frankly abnormal in level of membrane acetylcholinesterase and in complement sensitivity.

In search of the primary lesion in the PNH clone: membrane abnormalities

For over a century the search for the intrinsic red cell defect responsible for the increased complement sensitivity of PNH cells was unsuccessful. Until 1982 the only abnormality found was a marked decrease or absence of the membrane enzyme acetylcholinesterase (AchE), as determined by enzyme assay on haemolysates (De Sandre et al, 1956, Auditore and Hartmann, 1959) or by a cytochemical stain (Perona et al, 1965). Recently, the absence of AchE from PNH cells was confirmed quantitatively by flow cytofluorimetric analysis using an anti-AchE monoclonal antibody (Dockter and Morrison, 1986), but there is no obvious link between AchE activity and complement hypersensitivity and the role of AchE in red cells is unknown. Another enzyme abnormality, deficiency of alkaline phosphatase, was reported in granulocytes from PNH patients by Lewis and Dacie (1965).

Recently attention has been focused on membrane proteins which regulate complement activity on the cell surface. At least three distinct molecules have been identified. Two of them decrease the formation and the stability of C3 convertase on cell surface. One is a 250 kDa protein called C3b receptor, (CR1; Fearon, 1980); the other is a 70 kd protein called decay accelerating factor (DAF) (Nicholson-Weller et al, 1982). Other proteins have recently been found which inhibit the lytic action of the complement terminal complex. One is 80 kDa in size and has been called homologous restriction factor (HRF; Zalman et al, 1987); another is 65 kDa, named C8-binding protein (C8bp; Shin et al, 1986). All these proteins have been purified and specific antibodies are available. In the last 3 years, the following points have been established:

1. CR1 is present on PNH cells (Nicholson-Weller et al, 1983; Roberts et al, 1985). In one study it was found to be decreased in the blood of PNH subjects but both normal and PNH cells were equally affected indicating a secondary deficiency rather than a primary defect of the PNH clone (Medof et al, 1987).
2. DAF is absent or greatly reduced on PNH cells although it is normal on the normal red cells of PNH patients (Nicholson-Weller et al, 1983; Pagburn et al, 1983).
3. HRF and C8bp were not detected on red cells from PNH patients carrying the most severe abnormality (PNH-III cells: Hansch et al, 1987; Zalman et al, 1987).

Since all of the above molecules protect cells from complement lysis, deficiency of any of them might be associated with complement hypersensitivity. DAF deficiency will produce increased C3 convertase activity while HRF or C8bp deficiency is associated with higher sensitivity to the direct lytic activity of C5b-9. Deficiency of DAF in PNH patients has been demonstrated not only in red cells but also in a proportion of granulocytes and platelets (Nicholson-Weller et al, 1985), in keeping with the accepted notion that these cells share the PNH abnormality. In some but not all patients a proportion of DAF negative cells was found among lymphocytes (Kinoshita et al, 1985), indicating that in these cases a cell earlier than a myeloid progenitor may have been the target of the PNH mutation. By the use of immunoprecipitation (Chow et al, 1985), laser flow cytometry (Kinoshita et al, 1985), blotting (Hansch et al, 1987) and immunoradiometric assays (Medof et al, 1987) with appropriate monoclonal antibodies, it has been shown that not only is the activity of these proteins deficient, but the proteins themselves are absent or greatly reduced. Complement resistance was restored, at least partially, by insertion on cell membrane of purified proteins (Davitz et al, 1986; Zalman et al, 1987). Very recently, a fourth glycoprotein has been found deficient on PNH cells: the lymphocyte function-associated antigen 3 (LFA-3), a cell surface molecule of 45–70 kDa that is a ligand for CD2 (the E-rosette receptor; Selvaraj et al, 1987). It is still unknown if this molecule has any role on erythrocyte (or its precursor) surface, but it is certainly important for T-lymphocyte activation and its deficiency might explain certain aspects of immune function impairment in at least some PNH patients (Vellenga et al, 1981; Yoda and Abe, 1985).

At first sight the discovery of multiple membrane abnormalities (Table 3) does not fit well with the notion that PNH arises from the clonal expansion of a mutant cell, which would be expected to have a single primary lesion. Moreover, a somatic mutation is expected to affect only one of the two genes on homologous chromosomes. If the gene hit was the structural gene for one of the proteins mentioned above, a mutation should not lead to complete absence of synthesis of one, much less of several proteins. What do AchE, alkaline phosphatase, DAF, HRF, C8bp and LFA-3 have in common to explain their concomitant reduction or absence on PNH cells? Interestingly, it turns out that at least four of them (HRF and C8bp have not yet been tested) do share a unique chemical similarity, namely that they are bound to the outer surface of the cell through a phospholipid anchorage system (Low and Zilversmit, 1980; Low et al, 1986; Figure 2). The primary defect might be in the mechanism of anchoring (or of keeping anchored) these molecules to the cell surface. By using purified molecules it has been possible to bind firmly a suboptimal amount of both DAF (Medof et al, 1985) and C8bp

Table 3. Membrane abnormalities in PNH cells.

Deficiency in	Red cells	Granulocytes	Platelets	Lymphocytes
Ache	Yes	NA	NA	NA
Alkaline phosphatase	NA	Yes	NA	NA
DAF	Yes	Yes	Yes	Sometimes
HRF/C8bp	Yes		NA	
LFA-3	Yes	Partial*		

NA = not applicable because the molecule is not actually present on this type of cells from normal subjects.
* It has been suggested that LFA-3 is present in two forms on cell membrane; only one of them is bound via phosphatidylinositol. This form, which is impaire in PNH, is predominant on red cells, while granulocytes show predominantly the other one (Selvaray et al, 1987).
For references, see text.

(Zalman et al, 1987) to PNH cells, thus partially restoring resistance to complement lysis. It has also been shown that this type of molecule can be released from the surface of several types of cells by phosphatidylinositol-specific phospholipase C (Davitz et al, 1986). Preliminary unpublished data of Nussenzweig and Luzzatto indicate that PNH patients have increased amounts of free DAF molecules in the serum.

Although the primary lesion on PNH cells remains unknown, a working hypothesis can be formulated that the mutated gene encodes a product either required for processing the above-mentioned membrane proteins prior to apposition of the glycolipid anchor or for the synthesis of the glycolipid moiety itself. Such a model would confront the paradox of a single lesion causing a multitude of defects.

It is also possible that there is heterogeneity in the genetic lesion giving rise to the PNH phenotype. This may help to explain why some character-istics of the PNH clone may vary from one patient to another and why, in rare cases, more than one PNH population may coexist in the same patient. Indeed, there is now convincing evidence that PNH populations differing in

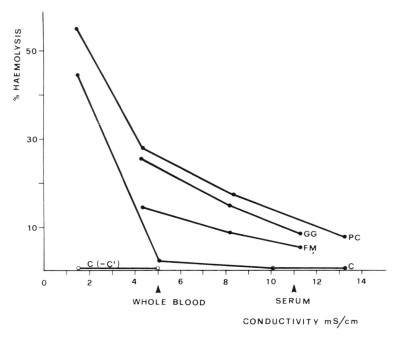

Figure 2. Haemolysis in the Ham test is a function of ionic strength. Red cells from three patients (PC, GG and FM) and a normal control (C) were tested against fresh compatible sera dialysed against iso-osmotic solutions of variable ionic strength containing Ca^{2+} (1 mmol/l) and Mg^{2+} (1 mmol/l). The electrical conductivity of the medium (abscissa) is a measure of the ionic strength. C (–C') = normal red cells tested with heat inactivated acid serum. Arrows indicate conductivity values corresponding to those of undialysed serum (conventional Ham test) and whole blood (presumably mimicking more closely in vivo conditions).

functional characteristics also differ in their molecular abnormalities. For instance, although both PNH-II and PNH-III cells lack DAF on their membrane, only PNH-III cells also bear the additional deficiencies of HRF and C8bp which lead to damage by C5-9 (Medof et al, 1987). The majority of patients possess either one or other abnormal cell type (single mutant clone) but in a few cases both PNH-II and PNH-III are present in the same patient, suggesting the presence of two mutant clones, one of which may conceivably have arisen through a second mutation in a cell belonging to the original PNH clone.

The size of the PNH clone

The size of the PNH clone might be assessed by simply measuring the percentage of cells lysed in one of the Ham-type diagnostic tests, but a number of errors are inherent in such an approach. Firstly, many PNH cells have been destroyed in vivo so the size of the clone will be underestimated. Secondly, various tests may give different results in the same patient, according to their sensitivity and specificity. Thirdly, it is not easy to reproduce in vitro all the conditions occurring in vivo and there is a risk either of measuring artefactual abnormalities or of missing a proportion of abnormal cells.

Several factors influence the result of the Ham test. The amount of lysis depends upon the potency of the serum (in other words, different results are obtained using sera from different donors), upon the pH and upon other experimental conditions, some of them usually ignored or unknown. The authors analysed the influence of ionic strength on the Ham test. The ionic strength of whole blood is much lower than that of plasma or serum, because the red cells, by immobilizing a cloud of ions around their negatively charged surface, reduce the availability of ions in the liquid phase. Several molecular interactions with cell membrane behave differently in whole blood compared to plasma or serum (Rotoli et al, 1987). Fresh human sera were dialysed to various ionic strengths using buffers composed of mixtures of iso-osmotic glucose (very low ionic strength) and iso-osmotic NaCl (high ionic strength; Rotoli et al, 1982b). When these dialysed sera were used to perform the Ham test, an inverse correlation between degree of haemolysis and serum conductivity (which is a measure of the ionic strength) was found in a number of PNH patients. As ionic strength decreased, the proportion of cells lysed increased. The percentage of red cells lysed at a conductivity corresponding to that of whole blood was three times greater than that obtained in the regular Ham test (Figure 3). At extremely low ionic strength even a portion of normal red cells underwent lysis in acidified serum. From this study we inferred that:

1. The conventional Ham test may underestimate the proportion of abnormal red cells.
2. A very mild PNH-like abnormality sufficient to cause haemolysis in vivo might not be detected by the conventional Ham test. Perhaps a more sensitive test in low ionic strength might reveal more frequently the PNH abnormality, e.g. in aplastic patients.
3. Lysis by activated complement is probably a physiological phenomenon that may affect normal red cells, perhaps the oldest ones.
4. The anaemia of PNH patients, by increasing whole blood conductivity, might effect some protection against haemolysis. Thus, as already mentioned, exacerbation of haemolysis following transfusion or iron replacement might be explained by the lower blood ionic strength associated with a higher haematocrit.

A better estimation of the size of the PNH clone could be obtained by in vitro cultures, although the method is not simple.

Progenitor cell cultures

Both quantitative and qualitative aspects of haemopoiesis in PNH patients have been investigated by in vitro cultures of progenitor cells, especially those giving rise to erythroid colonies. In the majority of patients a reduced number of erythroid colonies was found when peripheral blood or bone

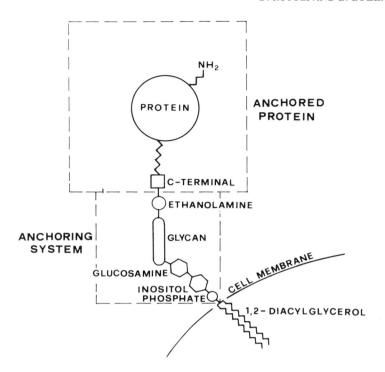

Figure 3. Diagram of the anchorage of protein molecules on the outer surface of cell membranes through a phosphatidylinositol covalent bridge (modified from Low et al, 1986). Besides DAF, AchE, alkaline phosphatase and LFA-3 (mentioned in the text), other proteins using this anchorage system include the Thy-1 glycoprotein in thymocytes and the variant surface glycoprotein in *Trypanosoma brucei*. In the last case, and perhaps in others, the functional significance of this anchorage system is that the surface protein can be rapidly shed by cleavage of the phosphate–glycerol bond by a specific phospholipase.

marrow-derived mononuclear cells were plated in a semisolid medium containing erythropoietin. In the bone marrow BFU-Es were more affected than CFU-E (Urabe and Fujioka, 1982). Peripheral blood BFU-Es were especially reduced, with complete absence of growth in a substantial number of cases. In seven PNH patients we found a tenfold reduction in circulating erythroid progenitors compared to normal age-matched subjects (Rotoli et al, 1982a). These data were then extended (Figure 4) and confirmed by other groups (Moore et al, 1982). The yield of erythroid colonies correlates with some clinical and haematological parameters; the more intense the anaemia and the more marked the aplastic character of PNH, the less the growth of colonies. Granulocyte colonies are also decreased in PNH patients (Tumen et al, 1980).

In vitro cultures have also helped to confirm the coexistence of normal and PNH progenitor cells, and to define the nature of some of the abnormalities

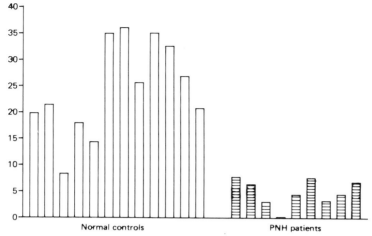

Figure 4. Reduced growth of erythroid colonies (BFU-E) from peripheral blood mononuclear cells of PNH patients, compared to normal subjects. Experimental conditions: culture in semisolid medium (methylcellulose 0.8%); erythropoietin 2 u/ml; cell concentration 5 × 10^5/ml; scoring on 13th day. Vertical axis: colonies/plate.

of the PNH clonal population. In brief, the following points were established:

1. By micromanipulation followed by cytochemical stain for AchE, two types of erythroid colonies (BFU-E) were found in PNH patients, one strongly positive and the other negative (Figure 5). The negative colonies were predominant. No negative colonies were ever detected in normal subjects (Rotoli et al, 1984).
2. Using a miniature Ham test, in which lysis in acidified fresh serum of a few cells from a single colony could be measured by release of radio-activity from colonies metabolically labelled with ^{3}H-leucine, we found two types of erythroid colonies from PNH patients, one of them highly sensitive to complement (Figure 6). When single colonies were split into two parts, one stained for AchE and the other tested by miniature Ham test, AchE-negative colonies invariably correlated with complement-hypersensitive colonies (Rotoli et al, 1984).
3. In an immunoradiometric assay using a mixture of three monoclonal anti-DAF antibodies (provided by Dr V. Nussenzweig), pooled erythroid cells grown from a PNH patient showed about 50% reduction in DAF when compared to erythroid cells grown from a normal subject (Rotoli et al, 1986). However, no single colonies totally lacking DAF were observed, and the distribution of DAF content on individual colonies was not bimodal. Since many of the colonies were PNH colonies, these data suggest that DAF is synthesized by PNH erythroid cells, and subsequently lost during their maturation.

In this respect, it is not yet clear at what stage in erythroid cell maturation the phenotypic expression of the PNH defect first appears. While it is known

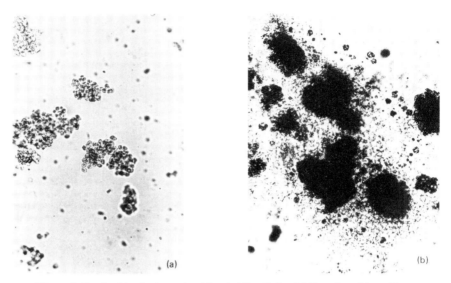

Figure 5. Erythroid colonies stained for AchE activity. **(a)** Negative; **(b)** positive.

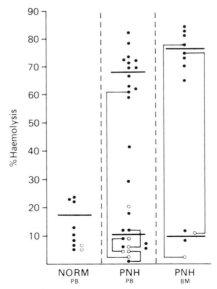

Figure 6. Evidence that erythroid colonies from a PNH patient are of two kinds, normally sensitive or hypersensitive to acid serum lysis (from Rotoli et al, 1984, with permission). Single bursts were assayed in fresh acidified serum (●) or in heat-inactivated acidified serum (○), and lysis was measured as ^{3}H-leucine-Hb release. In order to prove the specificity of the test, a number of bursts were split and both halves of the same colony were tested with fresh and inactivated serum respectively (vertical lines). Horizontal bars represent the mean for each group of data. NORM = normal control; PB = peripheral blood BFU-E; BM = bone marrow BFU-E.

that PNH normoblasts and myelocytes are hypersensitive to complement lysis, as demonstrated by ^{59}Fe and myeloperoxidase release respectively (Tumen et al, 1980), conflicting results concern the complement-sensitivity of more immature progenitor cells. Dessypris et al (1983) reported that the exposure of erythroid and myeloid progenitors to complement in a low ionic strength medium (sucrose test) caused a marked decrease in the number of colonies obtainable; similar results were obtained by the same group with respect to megakaryocytic colonies (Gleaton et al, 1986). By contrast, in unpublished experiments performed in 1980, we plated peripheral blood mononuclear cells from three PNH patients before and after treatment with acid serum (Ham), and we could not find any difference in the number of colonies obtained, indicating that erythroid progenitors are resistant to complement lysis. More recent experiments carried out by Moore et al (1985) seem to support our data. DAF-positive mononuclear cells from a PNH patient, sorted by a fluorescence-activated cell sorter using an anti-DAF antiserum, gave rise to erythroid colonies that were regarded as PNH because they had low DAF. Thus, it seems that although predetermined at a very early level, the PNH defect becomes apparent relatively late during differentiation.

A hypothetical model on the growth of the PNH clone and its relationship to aplastic anaemia

While it is widely accepted that the PNH cell population results from the expansion of a mutant clone, it is not immediately obvious why a 'diseased' clone should have the ability to displace normal haemopoiesis. A relative growth advantage must be postulated: either PNH cells are growing abnormally fast, or the normal haemopoietic cell growth is slowed down. The fact that most patients have hypoplastic bone marrow and a reduced number of haemopoietic progenitors clearly favours the second alternative; and both mechanisms could operate.

Because the pathogenesis of acquired aplastic anaemia is itself unknown, it is difficult and probably unwise to speculate about mechanisms. However, it is conceivable that the maturation of normal cells is hindered by some factor to which PNH cells are resistant. As a result, normal haemopoiesis will be reduced or even abolished, while the PNH clone thrives. An extreme example is seen in aplastic patients who develop PNH during the course of their disease. The growth advantage of PNH clones might lie in the absence of yet another molecule sharing the glycolipid anchoring system. The lack of LFA-3 is an example of a signal molecule involved in the set of abnormalities of PNH cells.

A somewhat fanciful model is illustrated in Figure 7. A PNH clone arising in a normal subject has no chance of emerging if haemopoiesis is normal (Figure 7a); instead, it will become manifest if the normal haemopoiesis is depressed (Figure 7b). Since the cause for reduced haemopoiesis may be quite independent of the development of the PNH clone, PNH may appear at any time during the course of the hypoplastic disease (Figure 7c). Finally, the PNH clone may become exhausted, showing a clinical sequence of PNH

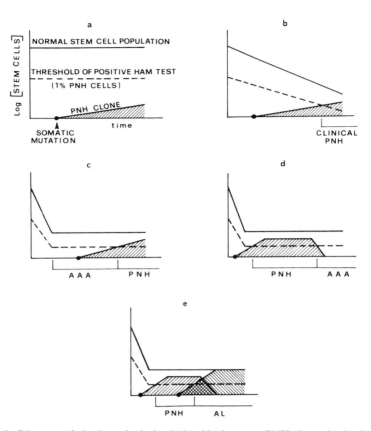

Figure 7. Diagram of the hypothetical relationship between PNH, hypoplastic disorders (acquired aplastic anaemia; AAA) and acute leukaemia (AL). **(a)** 'Silent' PNH: a clone with the PNH abnormality might be present in many normal subjects but it cannot be detected as long as the rest of the bone marrow is normal. **(b)** 'Typical' PNH: the PNH clone becomes detectable because the rest of the bone marrow is depressed **(c)** Aplastic anaemia with subsequent 'development' of PNH: the only difference from **(b)** is that the PNH clone has become detectable only after acquired aplastic anaemia was already clinically apparent. **(d)** PNH 'evolving' into aplastic anaemia: essentially a later stage of **(b)**, due to the fact that the PNH clone eventually becomes exhausted, because a single stem cell can only undergo a finite number of divisions. **(e)** PNH terminating in acute leukaemia. The leukaemogenic mutation (second dot) might take place in a normal stem cell (PNH followed by leukaemia) or within the PNH clone itself, in which case the leukaemic cells will bear the PNH defect (see text). In either case it may be impossible to obtain a remission without bone marrow transplantation, because there will be little or no bone marrow that can regenerate.

terminating in aplastic anaemia (Figure 7d). Another somatic mutation leading to a neoplastic transformation (e.g. acute leukaemia) may also occur independently of the previous mutation, causing a second haematopoietic disorder and possibly replacing the original PNH clone (Figure 7e). The second mutation may also arise from within the PNH clone. A recent report of Devine et al (1987) is probably an example of this event. Blast cells from a PNH patient who developed acute myeloblastic leukaemia were found to lack DAF, both by flow fluorocytometric analysis and by immunoblotting. Further studies probably on the same patient (Stafford et al, 1987) showed that DAF-negative blasts had normal DAF gene and mRNA transcripts, again indicating that the PNH defect has nothing to do with DAF synthesis.

TREATMENT

At present, no specific treatment is available for PNH. Therapy is essentially supportive though a cure may be achieved in some cases by bone marrow transplantation.

Blood transfusion support

The need for red cell transfusions varies according to the severity of the disease and its activity. Filtered or washed red cells should be used to minimize white cell and platelet alloimmunization and subsequent immune reactions. Anaemia is usually well tolerated by PNH patients and many may not require any transfusion for months or even years if they are allowed to stay with an Hb level of 7.5–8 g/dl.

Iron and iron chelation

Both iron replacement and iron chelation may have to be considered when managing patients with PNH. In the haemolytic form, recurrent haemoglobinuria and persistent haemosiderinuria often produce iron deficiency. Oral or even parenteral iron supplementation is needed in these patients. By contrast, in the aplastic form a regimen of regular red cell transfusion produces iron overload that may require desferrioxamine therapy.

Other drugs

Folic acid supplementation is indicated, as in any state of stressed haemopoiesis. A number of drugs have been used in an attempt to limit complement activation and/or stimulate haemopoiesis; they include heparin, tranexamic acid, androgenic steroids and prednisone (Rosse, 1982; Issaragrisil et al, 1987). However, the results have been erratic or questionable, and side-effects may be unacceptable.

Treatment of infectious complications must be prompt and energetic, especially if the patient is neutropenic, because infection may trigger an exacerbation of haemolysis.

Thrombotic complications are managed by the use of conventional drugs, including heparin, antiaggregating agents, and anticoagulants. There may be a role for thrombolytic agents, such as tissue plasminogen activator, especially in the acute stage of the most severe form of Budd–Chiari syndrome.

Splenectomy

Splenectomy may be considered for PNH patients with splenomegaly. This is a late finding usually following repeated transfusions in predominantly aplastic forms. If splenomegaly is marked, but especially if it is associated with increased red cell transfusion requirement and with evidence of hypersplenism in the way of leukopenia and thrombocytopenia, the beneficial effects of splenectomy may balance favourably the risk of the operation.

Bone marrow transplantation (BMT)

Allogeneic or syngeneic BMT is the only approach to a possible cure of PNH. At present, considering the relatively high morbidity and mortality associated with this procedure, BMT should probably be considered only when all of the following conditions are met: age of patient below 40; clinical and haematological picture of a severe aplastic anaemia; human leukocyte antigen (HLA)-identical sibling available.

The most compelling indication for BMT is life-threatening extreme thrombocytopenia and/or leukopenia. Less stringent indications for BMT will be applicable in the rare fortunate cases in which an identical twin is available as donor. It is hard to determine how many patients with PNH have been transplated so far, since some of them may have been included in series of severe aplastic anaemia. Small series or single cases have been reported (Storb et al, 1976; Hows et al, 1982; Gluckman et al, 1984; Szer et al, 1984); in some cases the donor was an identical twin (Fefer et al, 1976; Herskho et al, 1979; Champlin et al, 1984; Szer et al, 1984). In 1985 Antin et al collected eight cases in the literature and added four of their own cases.

Apart from its therapeutic effect, the outcome of BMT in PNH has provided some new information on the biology of the disease: since bone marrow repopulation was achieved following infusion of haemopoietic progenitors, no microenvironmental abnormality is likely to be responsible for PNH. Engraftment from identical twins was obtained in the absence of any cytotoxic treatment, and was followed by the disappearance of the PNH abnormality in at least two patients. Thus, normal stem cells seem to have a selective advantage over PNH cells, suggesting that the patient's own stem cells were abnormal. Lastly, heavy conditioning regimens (e.g. those designed to cause permanent marrow aplasia) do not seem to be necessary for allogeneic BMT in PNH patients.

These conclusions should be taken with caution, since BMT has only been carried out in aplastic patients, who may have their own progenitors exhausted; moreover, bone marrow infusion causes engraftment not only of haemopoietic progenitors, but also of a number of other different cell populations (e.g. lymphocyte subsets) that may co-operate in restoring a normal haemopoiesis.

CONCLUDING REMARKS

Having reviewed some of the advances in the clinical, pathophysiological and pathogenetic aspects of PNH, we cannot help feeling humbled by the consideration that, 50 years after the Ham test was introduced, the precise basis of this disease still defies full elucidation. However, the existing information and its practical implications can be briefly summarized as follows:

1. The PNH red cells belong to a single clone, presumably arisen through a somatic mutation in a stem cell. The PNH cell population is characterized by high sensitivity to lysis by activated complement, suggesting an abnormality in the membrane.
2. Membrane abnormalities which have been convincingly documented in PNH red cells include a marked reduction of various molecules (see Table 3) that share a common structural feature, namely a covalently linked phosphatidylinositol glycolipid anchor, suggesting that the primary lesion may consist in a failure in one of the steps in the pathway leading to the assembly of the anchorage structure.
3. Platelets and granulocytes also have membrane abnormalities, in keeping with the concept that the PNH somatic mutation has taken place in a multipotent stem cell. Qualitative changes in platelets may be conducive to their inappropriate activation, thus explaining the characteristic tendency to venous thrombosis which may be manifest in PNH patients even when they are thrombocytopenic, leading to potentially fatal complications such as the Budd–Chiari syndrome. In an analogous way, the documented and possibly other as yet unknown membrane changes in granulocytes may explain the abnormal susceptibility to infection of PNH patients which sometimes appears to be out of proportion to the degree of neutropenia.
4. The finding that normal (non-PNH) progenitor cells are regularly decreased in PNH patients indicates that, quite apart from the abnormality of the PNH clone itself, the bone marrow as a whole is affected. This is in keeping with the clinical observation of transition and overlap forms between PNH and acquired aplastic anaemia. An extreme view, reflected in the hypothetical model we have outlined (Figure 7), is that the PNH clone may actually be enabling some patients to survive a state of bone marrow failure which, in the absence of that clone, would amount to frank severe aplastic anaemia.
5. Very rarely, PNH cures itself, presumably because the PNH clone becomes extinct while bone marrow failure recovers spontaneously. Unfortunately, it is more common for the patient to succumb to an intercurrent complication, or the PNH clone to become extinct without bone marrow recovery (termination in severe aplastic anaemia). An

important therapeutic implication is that, if a suitable donor is available, bone marrow transplantation should be offered to the patient, probably more often than it has been hitherto.

From the biological point of view, PNH constitutes a unique example of a non-neoplastic clonal disease. The notion that a single clone may take over haemopoiesis largely or entirely is well founded in the experimental finding that lethally irradiated mice grafted with donor cells marked by transfected genes show repopulation of the bone marrow by a very limited number (two or three) of stem cells.

At the same time, the immediate challenge in PNH research is to identify the primary molecular lesion. Just as in genetic disorders, the somatic mutations giving rise to PNH may be heterogeneous. The known membrane abnormalities that we have reviewed point to a limited number of steps that may have been damaged by individual mutations, and therefore to a limited number of candidate genes. We do not presume to predict how soon one or more of them will be identified and cloned.

Acknowledgements

The authors are grateful to Ferdinando Frigeri and Vincenzo Martinelli for their help with the preparation of the manuscript, and to Aristide Della Porta for the original artwork.

REFERENCES

Antin JH, Ginsburg D, Smith BR et al (1985) Bone marrow transplantation for paroxysmal nocturnal hemoglobinuria: eradication of the PNH clone and documentation of complete lymphohematopoietic engraftment. *Blood* **66:** 1247–1250.

Aster RH & Enright SE (1969) A platelet and granulocyte membrane defect in paroxysmal nocturnal hemoglobinuria: usefulness for detecting platelet antibodies. *Journal of Clinical Investigation* **48:** 1199–1210.

Auditore JV & Hartmann RC (1959) Paroxysmal nocturnal hemoglobinuria. II. Erythrocyte acetylcholinesterase defect. *American Journal of Medicine* **27:** 401–410.

Brubaker LH, Essig LJ & Mengel CE (1977) Neutrophil life span in PNH. *Blood* **50:** 657–662.

Carmel R, Coltman CA, Yatteau RF & Costanza JJ (1970) Association of paroxysmal nocturnal hemoglobinuria with erythroleukemia. *New England Journal of Medicine* **283:** 1329–1331.

Champlin RE, Feig SA, Sparkes RS & Gale RP (1984) Bone marrow transplantation from identical twins in the treatment of aplastic anaemia: implication for the pathogenesis of the disease. *British Journal of Haematology* **56:** 455–463.

Chow FL, Telen MJ & Rosse WF (1985) The acetylcholinesterase defect in paroxysmal nocturnal hemoglobinuria: evidence that the enzyme is absent from the cell membrane. *Blood* **66:** 940–945.

Chow FL, Hall SE, Rosse WF & Telen MJ (1986) Separation of the acetylcholinesterase deficient red cells in paroxysmal nocturnal hemoglobinuria. *Blood* **67:** 893–897.

Cowall DE, Pasquale DN & Dekker P (1979) Paroxysmal nocturnal hemoglobinuria terminating as erythroleukemia. *Cancer* **43:** 1914–1916.

Craddock PR, Fehr J & Jacob HS (1976) Complement-mediated granulocyte dysfunction in paroxysmal nocturnal hemoglobinuria. *Blood* **47:** 931–939.

Crosby WH (1953) Paroxysmal nocturnal hemoglobinuria: relation of the clinical manifestations to underlying pathogenic mechanisms. *Blood* **8:** 769–812.

Dacie JV & Lewis SM (1972) Paroxysmal nocturnal haemoglobinuria: clinical manifestation, haematology, and nature of the disease. *Series Haematologica* **5:** 3–23.

Dameshek W (1969) Foreword and a proposal for considering paroxysmal nocturnal hemoglobinuria (PNH) as a 'candidate' myeloproliferative disorder. *Blood* **33:** 263–264.

Davitz MA, Low MG & Nussenzweig V (1986) Release of decay-accelerating factor (DAF) from the cell membrane by phosphatidylinositol-specific phospholipase C (PIPLC). *Journal of Experimental Medicine* **163:** 1150–1161.

De Sandre G, Ghiotto G & Mastella G (1956) L'acetilcolinesterasi eritrocitaria. II. Rapporti con le malattie emolitiche. *Acta Medica Patavina* **16:** 310–335.

Dessypris EN, Clark DA, McKee LC Jr & Krantz SB (1983) Increased sensitivity to complement of erythroid and myeloid progenitors in paroxysmal nocturnal hemoglobinuria. *New England Journal of Medicine* **309:** 690–693.

Devine DV, Gluck WL, Rosse WF & Weinberg JB (1987) Acute myeloblastic leukemia in paroxysmal nocturnal hemoglobinuria. Evidence of evolution from the abnormal paroxysmal nocturnal hemoglobinuria clone. *Journal of Clinical Investigation* **79:** 314–317.

Dockter ME & Morrison M (1986) Paroxysmal nocturnal hemoglobinuria erythrocytes are of two distinct types: positive or negative for acetylcholinesterase. *Blood* **66:** 540–543.

Fearon DT (1980) Identification of the membrane glycoprotein that is the C3b receptor of the human erythrocyte, polymorphonuclear leucocyte, B lymphocyte, and monocyte. *Journal of Experimental Medicine* **152:** 20–30.

Fefer A, Freeman M, Storb R et al (1976) Paroxysmal nocturnal hemoglobinuria and marrow failure treated by infusion of marrow from an identical twin. *Annals of Internal Medicine* **84:** 692–695.

Gleaton JH, Clark DA & Dessypris EN (1986) Increased sensitivity to complement (C') of megakaryocytic progenitors (CFU-M) in paroxysmal nocturnal hemoglobinuria (PNH). *Blood* **68(supplement 1):** 510.

Gluckman E, Marmont A, Speck B & Gordon-Smith EC (1984) Immunosuppressive treatment of aplastic anemia as an alternative treatment for bone marrow transplantation. *Seminars in Hematology* **21:** 11–19.

Ham TH & Dingle JH (1939) Studies on destruction of red blood cells. II. Chronic hemolytic anemia with paroxysmal nocturnal hemoglobinuria: certain immunological aspects of the hemolytic mechanism with special reference to serum complement. *Journal of Clinical Investigation* **18:** 657–672.

Hansch GM, Schonemark S & Roelcke D (1987) Paroxysmal nocturnal hemoglobinuria type III. Lack of an erythrocyte membrane protein restricting the lysis by C5b-9. *Journal of Clinical Investigation* **80:** 7–12.

Herskho C, Ho WG, Gale RP & Cline MJ (1979) Cure of aplastic anemia in paroxysmal nocturnal haemoglobinuria by marrow transfusion from identical twin: failure of peripheral leucocyte transfusion to correct marrow aplasia. *Lancet* **i:** 945–947.

Hirsch VJ, Neubach PA, Parker DM et al (1981) Paroxysmal nocturnal hemoglobinuria termination in acute myelomonocytic leukemia and reappearance after leukemic remission. *Archives of Internal Medicine* **141:** 525–527.

Holden D & Lichtman H (1969) Paroxysmal nocturnal hemoglobinuria with acute leukemia. *Blood* **33:** 283–286.

Hows JM, Palmer S & Gordon-Smith EC (1982) Use of cyclosporin A in allogenic bone marrow transplantation for severe aplastic anemia. *Transplantation* **33:** 382–386.

Issaragrisil S, Piankijagum A & Tang-Naitrisorana Y (1987) Corticosteroid therapy in paroxysmal nocturnal hemoglobinuria. *American Journal of Hematology* **25:** 77–83.

Katahira J, Aoyama M, Oshimi K, Mizoguchi H & Onada N (1983) Paroxysmal nocturnal hemoglobinuria terminating in Tdt-positive acute leukemia. *American Journal of Hematology* **14:** 79–87.

Kinoshita T, Medof ME, Silber R & Nussenzweig V (1985) Distribution of decay accelerating factor (DAF) in the peripheral blood of normal individuals and patients with paroxysmal nocturnal hemoglobinuria (PNH). *Journal of Experimental Medicine* **162:** 75–92.

Krause JR (1983) Paroxysmal nocturnal hemoglobinuria and acute non-lymphocytic leukemia. A report of three cases exhibiting different cytologic types. *Cancer* **51:** 2078–2082.

Kruatrachue M, Wasi P & Na-Nakorn S (1978) Paroxysmal nocturnal haemoglobinuria in Thailand with special reference to an association with aplastic anaemia. *British Journal of Haematology* **39:** 267–276.

Lewis SM & Dacie JV (1965) Neutrophil (leucocyte) alkaline phosphatase in paroxysmal nocturnal haemoglobinuria. *British Journal of Haematology* **11**: 549–556.

Lewis SM & Dacie JV (1967) The aplastic anaemia paroxysmal nocturnal haemoglobinuria syndrome. *British Journal of Haematology* **13**: 236–251.

Lewis SM, Szur L & Dacie JV (1960) The pattern of erythrocyte destruction in haemolytic anemia, as studied with radioactive chromium. *British Journal of Haematology* **6**: 122–139.

Low MG, Zilversmit DB (1980) Role of phosphatidylinositol in attachment of alkaline phosphatase to membranes. *Biochemistry* **19**: 3913–3918.

Low MG, Ferguson MAJ, Futerman AH & Silman I (1986) Covalently attached phosphatidylinositol as a hydrophobic anchor for membrane proteins. *Trends in Biochemical Sciences* **11**: 212–215.

Luzzatto L, Familusi JB, Williams CKO et al (1979) The PNH abnormality in myeloproliferative disorders: association of PNH and acute erythremic myelosis in two children. *Haematologica* **64**: 13–30.

Marchiafava E & Nazari A (1911) Nuovo contributo allo studio degli itteri cronici emolitici. *Policlinico (Sezione Medica)* **18**: 241–254.

Medof ME, Kinoshita J, Silber R & Nussenzweig V (1985) Amelioration of the lytic abnormalities of paroxysmal nocturnal hemoglobinuria with decay accelerating factor. *Proceedings of the National Academy of Sciences USA* **82**: 2980–2984.

Medof ME, Gottlieb A, Kinoshita T et al (1987) Relationship between decay accelerating factor deficiency, diminished achetylcholinesterase activity, and defective terminal complement pathway restriction in paroxysmal nocturnal hemoglobinuria erythrocytes. *Journal of Clinical Investigation* **80**: 165–174.

Micheli F (1931) Anemia (splenomegalia) emolitica con emoglobinuria-emosiderinuria tipo Marchiafava. *Haematologica* **12**: 101–106.

Moore JG, Humphries RK, Frank MM & Young N (1982) Profound deficiency of hematopoietic progenitor cells in paroxysmal nocturnal hemoglobinuria. *Blood* **60 (supplement 1)**: 39.

Moore JG, Frank MM, Muller-Eberhard HJ & Young NS (1985) Decay accelerating factor is present on PNH erythroid progenitors and lost during erythropoiesis in vitro. *Journal of Experimental Medicine* **162**: 1182–1192.

Moore JG, Humphries RK, Frank MM et al (1986) Characterization of the hemopoietic defect in paroxysmal nocturnal hemoglobinuria. *Experimental Hematology* **14**: 222–229.

Nicholson-Weller A, Burge S, Fearon DT, Weller PF & Austen KF (1982) Isolation of a human erythrocyte membrane glycoprotein with decay accelerating activity for C3 convertase of the complement system. *Journal of Immunology* **129**: 184–189.

Nicholson-Weller A, March SP, Rosenfields SI & Austen KF (1983) Affected erythrocytes of patients with paroxysmal nocturnal hemoglobinuria are deficient in the complement regulatory protein, decay accelerating factor. *Proceedings of the National Academy of Sciences USA* **80**: 5066–5070.

Nicholson-Weller A, Spicer DB & Austen KF (1985) Deficiency of the complement regulatory protein decay accelerating factor on membranes of erythrocytes, monocytes and platelets in paroxysmal nocturnal hemoglobinuria. *New England Journal of Medicine* **312**: 1091–1097.

Oni SB, Osunkoya BO & Luzzatto L (1970) Paroxysmal nocturnal hemoglobinuria: evidence for monoclonal origin of abnormal red cells. *Blood* **36**: 145–152.

Pagburn MK, Schreiber RD & Muller-Eberhard HJ (1983) Deficiency of an erythrocyte membrane protein with complement regulatory activity in paroxysmal nocturnal hemoglobinuria. *Proceedings of the National Academy of Science USA* **80**: 5430–5434.

Penny R & Galton DAG (1966) Studies on neutrophil function. II. Pathological aspects. *British Journal of Haematology* **12**: 633–645.

Perona G, Ghiotto G, Cortesi S et al (1965) A dual population of erythrocytes in paroxysmal nocturnal hemoglobinuria as demonstrated by histochemical detection of acetylcholinesterase. Proceedings of the 10th Congress of European Society of Haematology, p 388. Strasbourg.

Polli E, Sirchia G, Ferrone S et al (1973) Emoglobinuria parosistica notturna. Revisione critica. Milan: Edizioni Cilag–Chemie Italiana.

Resegotti L, Givone S (1962) Paroxysmal nocturnal haemoglobinuria. Report of a case in a 2 year old boy. *Acta Haematologica* **27**: 120–123.

Roberts WN, Wilson JG, Wong W et al (1985) Normal function of CR1 on affected erythrocytes of patients with paroxysmal nocturnal hemoglobinuria. *Journal of Immunology* **134:** 512–517.

Rosse WF (1982) Treatment of paroxysmal nocturnal hemoglobinuria. *Blood* **60:** 20–23.

Rosse WF & Dacie JV (1966) Immune lysis of normal and paroxysmal nocturnal hemoglobinuria (PNH) red blood cells. I. The sensitivity of PNH red cells to lysis by complement and specific antibody. *Journal of Clinical Investigation* **45:** 736–748.

Rosse WF & Gutterman LA (1970) The effect of iron therapy in paroxysmal nocturnal hemoglobinuria. *Blood* **36:** 559–565.

Rosse WF & Parker CJ (1985) Paroxysmal nocturnal haemoglobinuria. *Clinics in Haematology* **14:** 105–125.

Rosse WF, Logue GL, Adams J & Crookston JH (1974) Mechanism of immune lysis of the red cells in hereditary erythroblastic multi-nuclearity with a positive acidified serum test (HEMPAS) and paroxysmal nocturnal hemoglobinuria (PNH). *Journal of Clinical Investigation* **53:** 31–43.

Rotoli B, Robledo R & Luzzatto L (1982a) Decreased number of circulating BFU-Es in paroxysmal nocturnal hemoglobinuria. *Blood* **60:** 157–159.

Rotoli B, De Renzo A & Martinelli V (1982b) L'entità dell'emolisi acida nella EPN in relazione alla forza ionica del mezzo. *Haematologica* **67:** 801–802.

Rotoli B, Robledo R, Scarpato N & Luzzatto L (1984) Two population of erythroid cell progenitors in paroxysmal nocturnal hemoglobinuria. *Blood* **64:** 847–851.

Rotoli B, Formisano S & Luzzatto L (1986) Deficiency of decay accelerating factor (DAF) revealed by the use of monoclonal antibodies in erythroid colonies from patients with paroxysmal nocturnal hemoglobinuria (PNH). Proceedings of the International Symposium on Monoclonals and DNA probes in diagnostic and preventive medicine, Florence 1986. Abstract 117.

Rotoli B, Chiurazzi F, Buffardi S & Frigeri F (1987) Modulation of haemostatic molecular interations by red cells. In Barbui T et al (eds) *Cellular Blood Components in Haemostasis and Thrombosis Implications from Myeloproliferative Disorders*, pp 33–39. London: John Libbey.

Selvaraj P, Dustin ML, Silber R, Low MG & Springer TA (1987) Deficiency of lymphocyte function-associated antigen 3 (LFA-3) in paroxysmal nocturnal hemoglobinuria. Functional correlates and evidence for phosphatidylinositol membrane anchor. *Journal of Experimental Medicine* **166:** 1011–1025.

Shin ML, Hansch GM, Hu V & Nicholson-Weller A (1986) Membrane factors responsible for homologous species restriction of complement-mediated lysis: DAF operates at the C3/C5 convertase, while a second pronase sensitive factor(s) operates at C8 and C9 reaction. *Journal of Immunology* **136:** 1776–1782.

Sicigliano E, Rosenfield R, Cuttner J (1987) Aplastic anemia unresponsive to ATG with response to androgens and development of PNH. *Blood* **70 (supplement 1):** 190.

Sirchia G & Lewis SM (1975) Paroxysmal nocturnal haemoglobinuria. *Clinics in Haematology* **4:** 199–229.

Sirchia G, Ferrone S & Mercuriali F (1964) The action of two sulphydryl compounds on normal human red cells. Relationship to red cells of paroxysmal nocturnal hemoglobinuria. *Blood* **25:** 502–510.

Stafford HA, Weinberg JB, Rosse WF, Tykocinski ML & Medoff ME (1987) Intact decay accelerating factor (DAF) gene and mRNA transcripts in DAF negative blasts of acute myelogenous leukemia (AML) evolving in paroxysmal nocturnal hemoglobinuria (PNH). *Blood* **70 (supplement 1):** 930.

Storb R, Thomas ED, Welden PL et al (1976) Aplastic anemia treated by allogeneic bone marrow transplantation: a report on 49 cases from Seattle. *Blood* **48:** 817–841.

Strübing P (1882) Paroxysmal hemoglobinuria. *Deutsche Medizinische Wochenschrift* **8:** 1–14.

Szer J, Peeg HJ, Whitherspoon RP et al (1984) Long term survival after marrow transplantation for paroxysmal nocturnal hemoglobinuria with aplastic anemia. *Annals of Internal Medicine* **101:** 193–195.

Tumen J, Kline LB, Fay JW et al (1980) Complement sensitivity of paroxysmal nocturnal hemoglobinuria bone marrow cells. *Blood* **55:** 1040–1046.

Urabe A & Fujioka S (1982) Erythroid progenitors in paroxysmal nocturnal haemoglobinuria. *British Journal of Haematology* **50:** 295–298.

Vellenga E, Mulder NH & The TH (1981) Immunological dysfunction in paroxysmal nocturnal haemoglobinuria. *Clinical and Laboratory Haematology* **3:** 307–316.

Yoda Y & Abe T (1985) Deficient natural killer (NK) cells in paroxysmal nocturnal haemoglobinuria (PNH): studies of lymphoid cells fractionated by discontinuous density gradient
centrifugation. *British Journal of Haematology* **60:** 669–675.

Zalman LS, Wood LM, Frank MM & Muller-Eberhard HJ (1987) Deficiency of the homologous restriction factor in paroxysmal nocturnal hemoglobinuria. *Journal of Experimental
Medicine* **165:** 572–577.

8

Fanconi anaemia—constitutional, familial aplastic anaemia

E. C. GORDON-SMITH
T. R. RUTHERFORD

In 1927 Fanconi, in Switzerland, described a family in which three brothers developed aplastic anaemia. In addition to the pancytopenia they had microcephaly, abnormal skin pigmentation, internal strabismus and genital hypoplasia (Fanconi, 1967). Further families were described which led to the recognition of a particular inherited disorder, named after Fanconi, in which delayed onset of aplastic anaemia was associated with somatic and skeletal abnormalities which follow a definite pattern. The haematological features are characterized by a relentless progression to severe aplastic anaemia and the high incidence of acute non-lymphoblastic leukaemia in affected patients.

CLINICAL FEATURES

The typical patient with Fanconi's anaemia (FA) is readily recognized but the characteristic skin and skeletal abnormalities are not expressed in all patients. The most common findings are shown in Table 1.

Growth retardation

The birthweight is low in the majority of patients who developed FA compared with their normal siblings. Growth retardation occurs in about 75% of affected individuals (Gmyrek and Sylm-Rapoport, 1964) and many patients are presented to paediatricians for investigation of short stature. A hormonal cause for failure to grow has been sought but in most cases growth hormone levels are normal, though deficiency has occasionally been noted (Clarke and Weldon, 1975). The use of recombinant growth hormone in these patients may lead to an increase in acute leukaemia (Fisher et al, 1988; Watanabe et al, 1988). The failure is not always severe; most patients are between the first and tenth centile. In some families growth retardation is not a major feature, emphasizing the heterogeneity of the disorder (Duckworth-Rysiecki et al, 1984).

Table 1. Somatic abnormalities in Fanconi anaemia.

	Approximate incidence (%)
Low birthweight	55–60
Growth retardation	
Skeletal abnormalities	60
Thumbs	
Hands/wrists	
Forearms	
Microcephaly	50
Micro-ophthalmia	
Microstomia	
Skin pigmentation	75
Generalized hyperpigmentation	
Café au lait patches	
Depigmented spots	
Renal anatomical abnormalities	30
Horseshoe kidney	
Pelvic kidney	
Strabismus	25
Genital abnormalities	20
Cryptorchism	
Hypoplasia	
Mental retardation	20

Skeletal abnormalities

In classical cases the skeletal abnormalities of FA make patients readily recognizable (Figure 1a). Microcephaly, microphthalmia and small mouth and jaw give the patients an attractive and somewhat elfic appearance. Abnormalities of the hands are common, mostly affecting the thumbs. The thumb may be absent, rudimentary, triphalangeal or there may be absence of the first metacarpal (Figure 1b). Absence of the thumb may be associated with absence of the radius, with one or both sides being affected. Radiological changes in ossification centres or thinning of the phalanges may be noted (Endo et al, 1988).

Skin pigmentation

Café au lait patches of hyperpigmentation are characteristic in light-skinned patients and darker patches may be discerned in dark races. These patches are variable in size with somewhat irregular outlines, although not usually larger than about 4cm of maximum diameter. They occur most commonly on the trunk and back. Less marked but equally characteristic are small patches of depigmentation (Figure 1c). These are scattered small (0.5 cm) circular areas seen also mainly on the trunk and back.

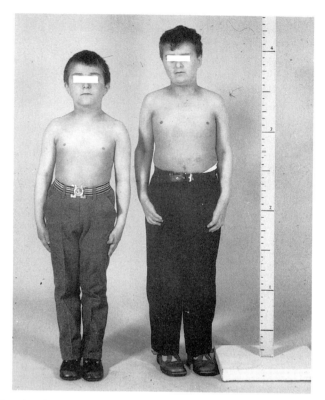

Figure 1a. Two brothers with Fanconi anaemia. Both had short stature, increased pigmentation, microcephaly and abnormal hands.

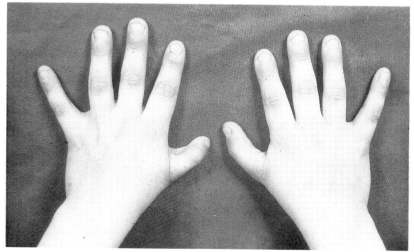

Figure 1b. Hands of a child with Fanconi anaemia showing dysplastic thumbs.

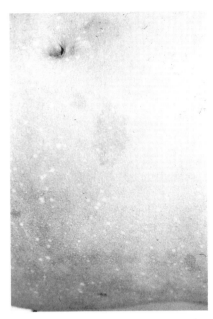

Figure 1c. Abdomen of a patient with Fanconi anaemia showing café au lait patches and depigmented spots.

Central nervous system

Mental retardation has been described but is not common and is not an inevitable consequence of the microcephaly. Strabismus is common. Hyperreflexia was described in the original family studied by Fanconi and is common, although often unremarked.

Urogenital abnormalities

Renal anatomical abnormalities are common, including horseshoe kidney and pelvic kidneys. The abnormal renal anatomy may lead to problems with reflux pyelonephritis. It is important to check the renal anatomy and function before embarking on bone marrow transplantation for these children so that appropriate modifications to drug therapy can be made.

In males genital hypoplasia and cryptorchism are common.

Other abnormalities

A number of other abnormalities have been reported in occasional families but it is difficult to be certain that they are part of the syndrome since consanguinity may lead to inheritance of other disorders. The abnormalities include deafness, atresia of the external auditory canal and atrophy of the spleen.

Haematological changes

At birth the blood count is normal. Pancytopenia develops insidiously and presents in most cases between the ages of 5 and 10 years (Gmyrek and Sylm-Rapoport, 1964). There is a group of patients in whom the pancyto-penia develops later during adolescence or even early adult life. It is possible that the genetic defect in these two groups is different (see below). The platelet count is the first to fall and patients often present with bruising. Anaemia develops but the granulocyte count is often well preserved in the early stages of the disease.

The bone marrow becomes progressively hypocellular once the pancyto-penia is noted. In the early stages, or before pancytopenia develops, the bone marrow may be hyperplastic with megaloblastic erythroid activity. As the pancytopenia develops the cellularity of the marrow decreases and in the end stages is indistinguishable from acquired aplastic anaemia. There is often a marked increase in macrophage activity; many macrophages show evidence of haemophagocytosis (Figure 2).

Patients with FA have increased risk of developing non-lymphoblastic leukaemia; perhaps as many as 10% of cases terminate in this way (Auerbach et al, 1982). Most cases are acute myeloblastic leukaemia but acute myelo-monoblastic, monoblastic and erythroleukaemia (Prindull et al, 1979) have been recorded. The disease may present as acute leukaemia (Auerbach et al, 1982) and there should be a high incidence of suspicion for FA in any child presenting with acute non-lymphoblastic leukaemia. The prognosis for the leukaemia is extremely poor since regeneration of the FA marrow is unlikely and the patients are sensitive to chemotherapeutic agents and

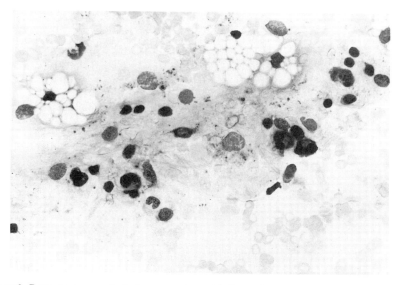

Figure 2. Bone marrow aspirate from a patient with Fanconi anaemia showing foamy macro-phages and haemophagocytosis.

radiation. It is important to identify those children presenting with acute leukaemia who have FA, not only because of the poor prognosis but so that other members of the family are examined and family counselling can be given.

The susceptibility to malignant change is mainly confined to the haemopoietic system although there has been suggestion that cancer of the gastrointestinal tract in particular is more common in relatives of these patients (Swift, 1971). Prolonged treatment with anabolic steroids induces a high incidence of hepatocellular carcinoma in these patients but there are no control groups to show whether this is a consequence of a genetic defect in DNA repair or the inevitable result of prolonged androgen therapy. Skin cancers are not increased in this group.

Chromosomal abnormalities

The characteristic feature of chromosomes from patients with FA is the increased occurrence of spontaneous chromosome damage (Schroeder,

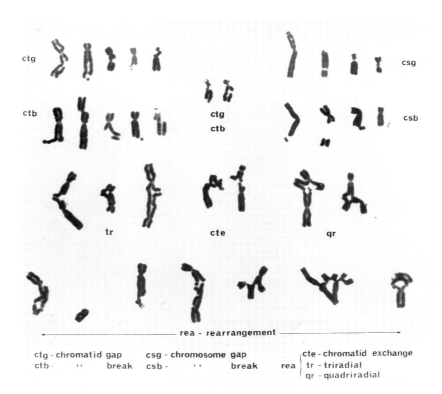

Figure 3. Chromosome analysis from cultured lymphocytes of a patient with Fanconi anaemia showing multiple chromatid anomalies (courtesy of Dr Murer-Orlando, Guy's Hospital, London).

1971) with an increased susceptibility to DNA crosslinking agents (see below). Typically the chromosomes exhibit an increase in chromosome gaps, breaks, constrictions, exchanges and translocations (Figure 3). These changes may be seen in lymphocytes or fibroblast cell lines. Clonal chromosome abnormalities are not part of FA but occur with malignant or premalignant change. Formal chromosome studies on haemopoietic cells are thus an important part of the investigation of a patient with FA.

GENETICS OF FA

FA is believed to be inherited as a mendelian autosomal recessive gene. This is supported by the high frequency of consanguineous marriage among parents of affected children. This view has been challenged on the basis of a number of observations: apparently non-mendelian ratios of affected to unaffected sibs, an apparent maternal age effect and a biased sex ratio (Miller and O'Reilly, 1984). However, Schroeder et al (1976), in a formal analysis of a large number of their own and published kindred, found no statistically significant deviation from strict mendelian inheritance.

FA has multiple developmental effects, which are quite variable between cases. This might suggest the existence of multiple gene loci for FA, or multiple alleles with different developmental defects at one locus. In fact neither explanation can be true in general, because large variation in the developmental abnormalities is also seen between affected members of the same family. This could be explained if there are other genes which modify the expression of FA, segregating in such families. An alternative explanation is that the developmental defects arise by stochastic events in small numbers of embryonic stem cells, and therefore are subject to large statistical variations.

The formal genetic data do not exclude the existence of more than one FA gene locus. Schroeder et al (1976) found a correlation between affected sibs in the age of onset of the anaemia. This could be partly due to environmental influences on the ascertainment of the disease but it has been tentatively suggested that early-onset and late-onset FA may belong to different complementation groups (Zakrzewski and Sperling, 1980). The formal method for demonstrating whether two individuals with a recessive condition have mutations in the same gene locus or at different loci is a complementation test. If two individuals have mutations at different loci, then their offspring after interbreeding will be normal, because the mutant gene from one parent will be complemented by a normal gene at that locus from the other parent, and vice versa. Since FA can be recognized in cultured cell lines by the cells' sensitivity to chromosome breakage and cell death in response to particular agents, a complementation test can be done by the methods of somatic cell genetics. Cultured cells from two individuals are fused and the hybrid cells tested to see if the defects in the two parental cell lines complement each other.

Complementation between FA cell lines was first reported by Zakrzewski and Sperling (1980). More recently Duckworth-Rysiecki et al (1985) began a

systematic study of complementation in FA by first isolating FA lympho-
blastoid cell lines carrying selectable mutations to aid in the isolation of cell
hybrids. In a series of well characterized hybrids they observed complementation of sensitivity to growth inhibition by mitomycin C (MMC), to
chromosome breakage induced by MMC, and to spontaneous chromosome
breakage, showing that there are at least two complementation groups and
therefore two gene loci responsible for FA.

FA and DNA repair

FA cells are believed to be defective in some aspect of DNA repair because
they are particularly sensitive to chromosome damage or inhibition of
growth by agents known to damage DNA. In 1975 Sasaki noted that while
FA cells were much more sensitive than normal cells to chromosome
damage induced by MMC, they were no more sensitive than normal cells to
a derivative, decarbamoyl mitomycin C (DCMMC). MMC is a bifunctional
reagent which can crosslink the two strands of the DNA helix, while
DCMMC is monofunctional and cannot generate interstrand crosslinks.
Sasaki therefore suggested that the primary defect in FA cells is in the repair
of DNA interstrand crosslinks. Since then a number of compounds which
can crosslink DNA strands have been shown to be particularly toxic to FA
cells; in some cases, closely related compounds which cannot crosslink DNA
strands were also studied, and found to be no more toxic to FA cells than to
normal cells (Sasaki and Tonomura, 1973; Auerbach and Wolman, 1976;
Berger et al, 1980; Ishida and Buchwald, 1982; Poll et al, 1985).

Various FA cell lines have also been shown to be more sensitive than
normal cells to agents which are not known to generate DNA interstrand
crosslinks. However this result has not been consistently found for FA cells
or cell lines from all cases, and the effect is generally quantitatively less than
for DNA crosslinking agents.

Fujiwata and co-workers (1977) directly studied the first 'unhooking' step
of DNA interstrand crosslink repair and found that FA cells were deficient
in this process. Others, however, have found contradictory results (Fornace
et al, 1979; Kaye et al, 1980; Sognier and Hittelman, 1983; Poll et al, 1984).
Interestingly, Sognier and Hittelman found that freshly isolated FA cell
lines were competent at crosslink repair, but lost this competence during
extended growth in culture.

Moustacchi et al (1987) have recently studied the repair of DNA
crosslinks by measuring the recovery of semi-conservative DNA replication
in cells treated with 8-methoxy-psoralen. They found that three FA cell lines
belonging to one complementation group recovered as rapidly as normal
cells, while in three cell lines of a different complementation group DNA
replication failed to recover. If their assay is indeed measuring crosslink
removal and if their results can be replicated with a larger number of FA cell
lines, then some of the contradictions noted above will be resolved.

Other DNA repair-related defects have been reported in FA cells including deficiency of DNA ligase activity (Hirsch-Kauffmann et al, 1978) and
defects in adenosine diphosphate ribosyl transferase (Schweiger et al, 1987).

It is not clear whether these defects are present in all FA cells or whether they are primary or acquired defects.

Superoxide metabolism in FA

Superoxide has been implicated in the generation of chromosome breakage by ionizing radiation. Nordenson (1977) cultured lymphocytes from FA patients in the presence or absence of superoxide dismutase (SOD) and catalase. She found that both SOD and catalase decreased the number of spontaneously occurring chromosome breaks. Joenje and co-workers (1978, 1979) measured the SOD activity directly in erythrocytes, and found that erythrocytes of FA patients had decreased activity compared to normal. They proposed that the primary defect in FA is in oxygen metabolism and not in DNA repair. Other groups have confirmed this decrease in SOD in FA erythrocytes (Okahata et al, 1980; Maveth et al, 1982) and lymphocytes (Yoshimitsu et al, 1984), although with one dissenting report (Scarpa et al, 1985). Others have also confirmed the protection of FA cells against both spontaneous and induced chromosome breakage by SOD, catalase and other antioxidants (Raj and Heddle, 1980; Nagasawa and Little, 1983; Dallapiccola et al, 1985b). Joenje et al (1981) have also shown that chromosome breakage in FA lymphocytes is sensitive to oxygen tension in culture.

How strong is the case for a primary defect in SOD or in superoxide metabolism? The decreases in SOD activity observed were mostly less than 50%, which seems unlikely for the direct effect of a homozygous recessive condition. Furthermore Gille et al (1987) have observed a case with decreased SOD in erythrocytes but higher than normal SOD activity in fibroblasts of the same patient. Raj and Heddle (1980) have argued that if the primary defect in FA cells is in oxygen metabolism, then they should show a much greater relative protection by antioxidants against chromosome breakage than should normal cells. In fact they found that although FA cells had higher levels of spontaneous and induced chromosome breakage, their relative protection by SOD was indistinguishable from that of normal cells.

It seems unlikely that there is a primary defect in oxygen metabolism in FA cells, but probable that superoxide metabolism is closely involved in the cellular pathology. It may be that the DNA of both normal and FA cells is receiving continual insults from intracellular superoxide or oxygen radicals, and that the normal cells are competent to repair the damage, while the FA cells are not. However, it is not clear how a hypothesis of oxygen damage to the DNA could be reconciled with the DNA crosslinking hypothesis of FA.

Prospects for cloning the FA genes

While the FA gene products are not known, it may still be possible to clone the FA genes by a cell selection strategy. FA cells are extremely sensitive to growth inhibition and killing by DNA crosslinking agents such as MMC. If FA cells were transfected with DNA from normal cells and then challenged with MMC, then the FA cells would be killed, except that any cell which had taken up and expressed the normal allele of the FA gene would be resistant to MMC and would grow. If the normal DNA used was not human DNA but mouse DNA, say, then the mouse DNA in the human cell could be distinguished by the presence of mouse repetitive DNA sequences. Using these, the mouse equivalent of the FA gene could be cloned from the transfected cells. Cloning of the human equivalent would then be straightforward.

This method has been used to clone DNA repair genes, but the experiment is far from trivial. First, the transfection efficiency of untransformed fibroblast cell lines is very low, although Diatloff-Zito et al (1986) have observed correction of FA cells' sensitivity to MMC after transfection with human DNA. There exists a simian virus 40 (SV40)-transformed FA cell line with a much elevated transfection efficiency (Duckworth-Rysiecki et al, 1986). When Buchwald et al (1987) transfected these cells with DNA from Chinese hamster ovary (CHO) cells they obtained MMC-resistant clones; however, these clones did not contain Chinese hamster DNA and presumably were genetic revertants. The mutations in FA may frequently be point mutations with a significant reversion frequency, and the reversion rate may even be increased in SV40-transformed cells.

Shaham et al (1987) have now reported the recovery of FA cells containing CHO DNA after DNA transfection and selection in the DNA crosslinking agent diepoxybutane. These cells are now good candidates for cloning of FA genes, although success will depend on the size of the genes, and the proximity of Chinese hamster repetitive DNA elements to the genes.

PATHOPHYSIOLOGY

Bone marrow failure seems to be a consequence of haemopoietic stem cell failure without any obvious change in the marrow stroma. Precursor cells are reduced in number commensurate with the peripheral blood pancytopenia and growth factor production is normal or increased. Precursor cell colonies appear normal in culture unless malignant or premalignant change has occurred. Lymphoblasts and fibroblasts grow in culture but may have decreased growth rates compared with normal subjects.

CLINICAL COURSE AND MANAGEMENT

In the great majority of patients the bone marrow failure progresses inexorably to complete aplasia unless the course is interrupted by the development of acute leukaemia. However, spontaneous recovery of blood count has been reported though it is not clear how often this occurs or whether it is more likely to occur in affected members of the same family. In these reported cases of spontaneous recovery improvement in the blood count has occurred mostly at the time of puberty.

Many patients—probably the majority—respond to treatment with anabolic steroids. Following the introduction of high-dose therapy, for example 2.5 mg/kg/day oxymetholone, the haemoglobin stabilizes and starts to rise

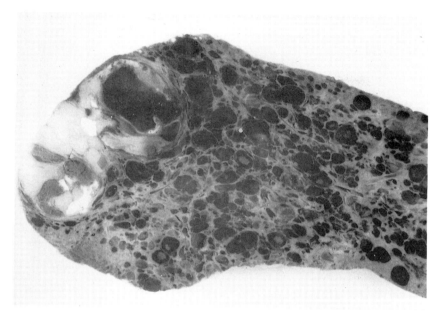

Figure 4. Section of liver from a patient with Fanconi anaemia who had received oxymetholone treatment for 4 years. Section shows multiple blood lakes (peliosis), hepatic and hepatocellular carcinoma on the left.

after about 6 weeks. The effect of the androgens is not only on the erythroid series but also there is usually improved platelet and granulocyte count. This improvement in blood count is achieved at considerable cost. The anabolic steroids produce inevitable virilizing effects which are particularly distressing in young children—not only girls but also boys. Apart from the changes in hair growth and sexual development the androgens frequently produce behavioural changes, making the children aggressive and irritable. Hepatotoxicity is almost inevitable after several months of treatment; rises in bilirubin and alkaline phosphatase are the first to be noted. Further changes develop with hyperplasia of hepatocytes and further structural changes include the development of peliosis hepatis and/or hepatocellular carcinoma (Figure 4). The carcinoma may be multicentric or a single tumour (Meadows et al, 1974). Regression of the tumour may occur after withdrawal of androgens although there may be relapse after some years of apparently being free from the disease. At present androgens may only be considered as a holding procedure until a suitable bone marrow donor can be found for transplantation.

ANTENATAL DIAGNOSIS

As with all inherited conditions, particularly those like FA with a poor prognosis, family counselling plays an important part in management. Antenatal diagnosis is now possible for FA (Auerbach et al, 1981, 1985, 1986; Dallapiccola et al, 1985a) and should be discussed urgently with parents of afflicted children. The characteristic chromosome instability is present in amniotic fluid cells and in fetal blood cells. Auerbach and colleagues (1986) have developed antenatal screening tests using the increased sensitivity of FA cells to diepoxybutane, initially using amniotic fluid cells and more recently chorionic villus cells in the first trimester. Fetal blood sampling and monitoring the effect of MMC on FA chromosome has also been used in prenatal diagnosis.

REFERENCES

Auerbach AD & Wolman SR (1976) Susceptibility of Fanconi's anemia fibroblasts to chromosome damage by carcinogens. *Nature* **261:** 494–496.
Auerbach AD, Adler B & Chaganti RSK (1981) Prenatal and postnatal diagnosis and carrier detection of Fanconi's anemia by cytogenetic method. *Pediatrics* **67:** 128–135.
Auerbach AD, Weiner MA, Warburton D et al (1982) Acute myeloid leukemia as the first hematologic manifestation of Fanconi anemia. *American Journal of Hematology* **12:** 289.
Auerbach AD, Sagi M & Adler B (1985) Fanconi anemia: prenatal diagnosis in 30 fetuses at risk. *Pediatrics* **76:** 794–800.
Auerbach AD, Zhang M, Ghosh R et al (1986) Clastogen induced chromosomal breakage as a marker for first trimester prenatal diagnosis of Fanconi anaemia. *Human Genetics* **73:** 86–88.
Berger R, Bernheim A, Le Coniat M et al (1980) Nitrogen mustard-induced chromosome breakage: a tool for Fanconi's anemia diagnosis. *Cancer Genetics and Cytogenetics* **2:** 269–274.
Buchwald M, Ng J, Clarke C et al (1987) Studies of gene transfer and reversion to mitomycin C resistance in Fanconi anemia cells. *Mutation Research* **184:** 153–159.
Clarke WL & Weldon MC (1975) Growth hormone deficiency and Fanconi's anemia. *Journal of Pediatrics* **86:** 814.
Dallapiccola B, Carbone LDL, Ferranti G et al (1985a) Monitoring of pregnancies at risk for Fanconi's anemia by chorionic villus sampling. *Acta Haematologica* **73:** 157–158.
Dallapiccola B, Porfirio B, McKini V et al (1985b) Effect of oxidants and antioxidants on chromosomal breakage in Fanconi anaemia lymphocytes. *Human Genetics* **69:** 62–65.
Diatloff-Zeto C, Papadopoulo D, Auerbeck D et al (1986) Abnormal response to DNA cross linking agents of Fanconi anemia. Fibroblasts can be corrected by transfection with normal human DNA. *Proceedings of the National Academy of Science* **83:** 7034–7038.
Duckworth-Rysiecki G, Hulten M, Mann J & Taylor AMR (1984) Clinical and cytogenetic diversity in Fanconi's anaemia. *Journal of Medical Genetics* **21:** 197–203.
Duckworth-Rysiecki G, Cornish K, Clarke CA et al (1985) Identification of two complementation groups in Fanconi anaemia. *Somatic Cell and Molecular Genetics* **11:** 35–41.
Duckworth-Rysiecki G, Toji L, Ng J et al (1986) Characterization of a simian virus 40-transformed Fanconi's anaemia fibroblast cell line. *Mutation Research* **166:** 207–214.
Endo M, Kaneko Y, Shikano T, Minami H & Chind J (1988) Possible association of human growth hormone treatment with an occurrence of acute myeloblastic leukemia with an inversion of chromosome 3 in a child with pituitary dwarfism. *Medical Pediatric Oncology* **16:** 45–47.
Fanconi G (1927) Familiare infantile periziosaartige Anämie (pernizioses Blutbild und Konstitution). *Zeitschrift für Kinderheilkunde* **117:** 257.
Fanconi G (1967) Familial constitutional panmyelopathy, Fanconi's anemia (FA) I. Clinical aspects. *Seminars in Hematology* **4:** 233.
Fisher DA, Job J-C, Preece M & Underwood LE (1988) Leukaemia in patients treated with growth hormone. *Lancet* **i:** 1159–1160.
Fornace AJ Jr, Little LB & Weichselbaum RR (1979) DNA repair in a Fanconi's anaemia fibroblast cell strain. *Biochimica Biophysica Acta* **561:** 99–109.

Fujiwata Y, Tatsumi M & Sasaki MS (1977) Cross-link repair in human cells and its possible defect in Fanconi's anaemia cells. *Journal of Molecular Biology* **113**: 635–649.

Gille JJP, Wortelbaer HM & Joenje H (1987) Antioxidant status of Fanconi anemia fibroblast. *Human Genetics* **77**: 28–31.

Gmyrek D & Sylm-Rapoport I (1964) Analysis of 129 reported cases of Fanconi's anemia. *Zeitschrift für Kinderheilkunde* **91**: 297.

Hirsch-Kauffmann M, Schweiger M, Wagner EF et al (1978) Deficiency of DNA ligase activity in Fanconi's anaemia. *Human Genetics* **45**: 25–32.

Ishida R & Buchwald M (1982) Susceptibility of Fanconi's anaemia lymphoblast to DNA cross-linking and alkylating agents. *Cancer Research* **42**: 4000–4006.

Joenje H, Eriksson AW, Frants RR et al (1978) Erythrocyte superoxide-dismutase deficiency in Fanconi's anaemia. *Lancet* **?**: 204.

Joenje H, Frants RR, Arwort F et al (1979) Erythrocyte superoxide dismutase deficiency in Fanconi's anaemia established by two independent methods of assay. *Scandinavian Journal of Clinical Laboratory Investigation* **39**: 759–764.

Joenje H, Arwert F, Eriksson AW et al (1981) Oxygen-dependence in Fanconi's anaemia. *Nature* **290**: 142–143.

Kaye J, Smith C & Hanawalt PC (1980) DNA repair in human cells containing photoadducts of 8 methoxypsoralen or Angelicin. *Cancer Research* **40**: 696–702.

Mavelli I, Ciriolo MR, Rotilio G et al (1982) Superoxide dismutase, glutathione peroxidase and catalase in oxidative hemolysis. A study of Fanconi's anaemia erythrocytes. *Biochemical and Biophysical Research Communications* **106**: 286–290.

Meadows AT, Haiman JL & Valdes-Dapena M (1974) Hepatoma associated with androgen therapy for aplastic anemia. *Journal of Pediatrics* **84**: 109.

Miller DR & O'Reilly J (1984) In Miller DR et al (eds) *Blood Diseases in Infancy and Childhood*, 5th edn, pp 542–554. St Louis: Mosby.

Moustacchi E, Papadopoulo D, Dratloff-Zito C et al (1987) Two complementation groups of Fanconi's anemia differ in their phenotypic response to a DNA-cross-linking treatment. *Human Genetics* **75**: 45–47.

Nagasawa M & Little JB (1983) Suppression of cytotoxic effect of mitomycin-C by superoxide dismutase in Fanconi's anaemia and dyskeratosis congenita fibroblast. *Carcinogenesis* **4**: 795–798.

Nordenson I (1977) Effect of superoxide dismutase and catalase on spontaneously occurring chromosome breaks in patient with Fanconi's anaemia. *Hereditas* **86**: 147–150.

Okahata S, Kobayashi Y & Usui T (1980) Erythrocyte superoxide dismatase activity in Fanconi's anaemia. *Clinical Science* **58**: 173–175.

Poll EHA, Arwort F, Joenje H et al (1985) Differential sensitivity of Fanconi's anaemia lymphocytes to the clastogenic action of CIS-diamminedichloroplatinum (II) and trans-diamminedichloroplatinum (II). *Human Genetics* **69**: 228–234.

Poll EHA, Arwert F, Kortbeck HT et al (1984) Fanconi anaemia cells are not uniformly deficient in unhooking of DNA interstrand cross links induced by mitomycin C or 8 methoxypsoralen plus UVA. *Human Genetics* **68**: 228–234.

Prindull G, Jentsch E & Hansmann I (1979) Fanconi's anaemia developing erythroleukaemia. *Scandinavian Journal of Haematology* **23**: 59.

Raj AS & Heddle JA (1980) The effect of superoxide dismutase, catalase and L-cysteine on spontaneous and on mitomycin C induced chromosomal breakage in Fanconi's and normal fibroblasts as measured by the micronucleus method. *Mutation Research* **78**: 59–66.

Sasaki MS (1975) Is Fanconi's anaemia defective in a process essential to the repair of DNA cross-links? *Nature* **257**: 501–503.

Sasaki MS & Tonomura A (1973) A high susceptibility of Fanconi's anemia to chromosome breakage by DNA cross-linking agents. *Cancer Research* **33**: 1829–1836.

Scarpa M, Rigo A, Momo F et al (1985) Increased role of superoxide ion generation in Fanconi's anaemia erythrocytes. *Biochemical and Biophysical Research Communications* **130**: 127–132.

Schroeder T (1971) Spontaneous chromosome breakage and high incidence of leukemia in inherited disease. *Blood* **37**: 96–112.

Schroeder TM, Tilgen D, Kruger J et al (1976) Formal genetics of Fanconi's anemia. *Human Genetics* **32**: 257–288.

Schweiger M, Auer B, Burtocher HJ et al (1987) DNA repair in human cells: biochemistry of the hereditary diseases Fanconi's anaemia and Cockayne syndrome. *European Journal of Biochemistry* **165:** 235–242.

Shaham M, Adler B, Ganguly S et al (1987) Transfection of normal human and Chinese hamster DNA corrects diepoxybutane-induced chromosomal hypersensitivity of Fanconi anaemia fibroblasts. *Proceedings of the National Academy of Science of the USA* **83:** 5853–5857.

Sognier MA & Hittelman WN (1983) Loss of repairability of DNA interstrand cross-links in Fanconi's anaemia cells with culture age. *Mutation Research* **108:** 383–393.

Sudharoan A & Heddle JA (1980) The effect of superoxide dismutase, catalase and L-cysteine on spontaneous and on mitomycin C induced chromosomal breakage in Fanconi's anaemia and normal fibroblasts as measured by the micronucleus method. *Mutation Research* **78:** 59–66.

Swift M (1971) Fanconi's anaemia and the genetics of neoplasia. *Nature* **230:** 371.

Watanabe S, Tsunematsu Y, Fujimoto J & Komiyama A (1988) Leukaemia in patients treated with growth hormone. *Lancet* **i:** 1159.

Yoshimitsu K, Kobayashi Y & Usui T (1984) Decreased SOD activity of erythrocytes and leukocytes in Fanconi's anaemia. *Acta Haematologica* **72:** 208–210.

Zakrzewski S & Sperling K (1980) Genetic heterogeneity of Fanconi's anaemia demonstrated by somatic cell hybrids. *Human Genetics* **56:** 81–84.

9

Bone marrow transplantation for Fanconi's anaemia

ELIANE GLUCKMAN

Fanconi's anaemia (FA) is an autosomal recessive inherited condition in which congenital malformations are associated with bone marrow failure (see Chapter 6). Multiple abnormalities of peripheral blood lymphocyte chromosomes are almost always present. In its natural course FA is usually fatal with death caused by progressive marrow aplasia or, less frequently, by development of acute leukaemia (Swift, 1976; Prindull et al, 1979). Bone marrow transplantation offers the potential for correction of the stem cell defect. In the past, the outcome of transplantation in these patients has been poor because of the severe prolonged toxicity of the pre-transplantation conditioning regimen and subsequent poor tolerance of graft versus host disease (GvHD; Gluckman et al, 1980). This poor tolerance to alkylating agents has been related to a DNA defect with increased chromosomal instability. Recently, efforts have been made to modify the conditioning regimen according to the cell sensitivity to alkylating agents and to irradiation.

ASSESSMENT OF THE DONOR

In FA it is essential to check that the donor is not also suffering from a clinically inapparent form of the disease by carrying out a cytogenetic analysis to determine whether he or she is healthy, a heterozygote or a homozygote for the FA gene. The type and frequency of chromosomal breaks vary markedly from patient to patient and in the same patient at different periods. For this reason, more sensitive tests have been described, which utilize the sensitivity of lymphocytes to DNA cross-linking agents. Berger et al (1980a) studied the effect of cyclophosphamide metabolites in FA and showed an augmentation of chromosomal breaks in FA lymphocytes when they were incubated with low concentrations of sera from a cyclophosphamide-treated patient. No effect was observed with comparable concentrations of cyclophosphamide on cells from parents of these patients or from controls. A similar effect was observed by Auerbach and colleagues (Auerbach et al, 1983). Nitrogen mustard added at a final concentration of $0.085\,\mu g/l$ after 1 day of culture of PHA-stimulated lymphocytes markedly increased the level of chromosome breakages in patients' cells. A clear distinction between patients and parents was possible allowing the detection of heterozygotes; nitrogen mustard added initially to the cultures significantly increased the sister chromatid exchange in FA heterozygotes when compared with normal controls. Auerbach described a hypersensitivity of FA cells to the blastogenic effect of diepoxy butane (DEB) (Auerbach, 1983). This test was used for the prenatal and postnatal diagnosis of FA. There was too much overlap between normal and FA heterozygote cells for accurate heterozygote detection.

RADIOSENSITIVITY IN FA

Lymphocytes from FA patients exposed to 1 Gy irradiation show a higher rate of chromosome breaks per cell than normal controls (Higurashi and Conen, 1971). An in vivo test of radiosensitivity and cell restoration as a predictor of the patients' response to irradiation for bone marrow transplantation conditioning has been described (Gluckman et al, 1983). The sensitivity of the skin to radiation was tested in two ways. In the first test, a measure of overall radiosensitivity, two areas of skin 15 mm in diameter on the anterior aspect of the thigh were irradiated with a 50 kV X-ray source at 0.5 Gy/s. One area received 8 Gy, the other 10 Gy. The skin was examined every 2 weeks for evidence of pigmentation (P) and desquamation (D). In a previous study of 20 normal controls, slight desquamation (D1) appeared between 30 and 40 days after irradiation (Dutreix et al, 1973). Cell repair was evaluated by comparing the reaction of the skin to a single dose of irradiation with the reaction after irradiation given in two equal fractions separated by an interval of 3–4 hours. Fractions of 4, 5, 6 or 7 Gy were given. Cell repair was considered normal if the skin reaction to a single 10 Gy dose was similar to that of a 2×6 Gy fractionated dose. Results are shown in Table 1. Twelve patients were studied before bone marrow transplantation

Table 1. Skin radiosensitivity test in Fanconi's anaemia.

Patient	Delay of reaction peak (days)	Reaction at 10 Gy	Repair	Number of abnormalities
SLA 87	55	D2	0	3
SLA 92	50	D2	0	3
SLA 97	40	D1	N	2
SLA 100	40	D2	N	2
SLA 101	50	D1	N	2
SLA 103	40	P2	N	2
SLA 116	40	D1	N	2
SLA 118	40	P	N	1
SLA 126	40	D2	N	2
SLA 134	40	D1	0	3
SLA 139	40	D1	N	2
SLA 148	40	D1	N	2

D = desquamation; P = pigmentation; 0 = no repair; N = normal repair.

for skin radiosensitivity for the purpose of predicting their reaction to the irradiation used for conditioning. The most constant abnormality was a delay in the peak skin reaction ranging from 40 to 55 days, in comparison with 30 days for 20 normal controls. This observation could be related to an increased transit time from the basal layer to the surface layer of the skin. The second abnormality observed in 10 patients was an increased sensitivity to a single dose of 10 Gy. The practical implication of the demonstration of an increased radiosensitivity is a proper adjustment of the irradiation dose given for conditioning. Absence of repair was demonstrated in only three cases. This finding can be related to the lack of sensitivity of the method or to the heterogeneity of the disease. Absence of repair implies that the relative protection expected from low dose rate or fractionated irradiation on tissues exhibiting rapid repair such as gut, mucosa and lung would not be possible. Because of these results, we have chosen to lower the irradiation dose from 6 to 5 Gy given in a single fraction at a mean dose rate of 10 cGy/min. The fields were calculated for complete protection of lungs, part of the liver, testicles in males, head and the inferior two-thirds of the legs.

The predictive value of the radiosensitivity remains to be demonstrated. In our series of patients, we did not find any correlation between the results of this test, the severity of the disease and the outcome of the graft.

SENSITIVITY TO ALKYLATING AGENTS

The sensitivity of FA cells to alkylating agents and in particular to DNA cross-linking compounds is well documented, and is discussed in greater detail in Chapter 8. Early clinical experience with high-dose cyclophosphamide suggested that this sensitivity to alkylating agents produced unacceptable side-effects (see below) and that modifications of the regimen used for acquired aplastic anaemia would be required for FA.

BONE MARROW TRANSPLANTATION

Conditioning regimen

Before 1980 in the Hôpital St Louis, five patients were conditioned with cyclophosphamide (100–200 mg/kg) given over 4 days. Detailed results are given in Table 2. Only one patient became a long-term survivor. Nine years after transplant she has a normal growth with signs of puberty. Her blood counts are normal and her chromosomal analysis shows the absence of abnormal chromosomal breaks (Berger et al, 1980b). The other patients died early after bone marrow transplantation. They all had toxic complications related to cyclophosphamide, namely haemorrhagic cystitis, cardiac failure, fluid overload, mucositis and intestinal haemorrhages, always associated with an early take and severe grade IV graft versus host disease (GvHD).

Table 2. Bone marrow transplant results after conditioning with cyclophosphamide 100–200 mg/kg.

Patient	Age	Sex	Take	A GvHD grade	Chronic GvHD	Survival
SLA 22	7	F	+	IV	0	>7 years A/W
SLA 31	11	M	+	IV	NE	+ 40 days GvHD
SLA 35	11	M	+	IV	NE	+ 48 days GvHD
SLA 44	10	F	+	IV	NE	+ 48 days GvHD
SLA 50	7	F	+	III	NE	+ 150 liver failure

A GvHD = acute graft versus host disease; NE = non-evaluable; A/W = alive and well.

These results prompted us to modify the conditioning according to in vitro tests of lymphocyte sensitivity to cyclophosphamide and to in vivo tests of radiosensitivity.

The new conditioning was similar to the one currently used in our unit for conditioning non-constitutional aplastic anaemia but the doses of chemo-radiotherapy were decreased.

In non-constitutional aplastic anaemia, cyclophosphamide 50 mg/kg i.v. was given on days −6, −5 and −4 and 6 Gy thoracoabdominal irradiation on day −1 (Gluckman et al, 1983). In FA we reduced the dose of cyclophosphamide to 5 mg/kg i.v. on days −6, −5, −4 and −3. As the radiosensitivity test did not seem to give any guidelines for dose reduction for an individual patient, we chose to decrease the dose from 6 to 5 Gy in one single dose at the mean dose rate of 6 cGy/min. The field involved the neck, trunk, upper part of the thigh and arms, with total shielding of the lung and the right part of the liver. The dose was not fractionated because of the poor benefit expected in this category of patients affected by a DNA repair defect.

Cyclosporin was given as prophylaxis for GvHD from day −1 to at least day 180 after transplantation. The initial dose was given according to a preliminary individual pharmacokinetic study (radioimmunoassay) in order to obtain a cyclosporin plasma level of 100 ng/ml. Subsequently, the dose of cyclosporin was adjusted to the results of weekly measurements of cyclosporin plasma levels and to blood urea and creatinine levels (Gluckman et al, 1984a).

Patients

The mean age at transplantation was 11.5 years (range 5–19). All patients had typical malformations associated with FA, but in three patients they were limited to few café au lait spots. Two patients had an affected sibling and in five other patients, the family history revealed cases of early infant deaths, malformations, aplasia or leukaemia. In three families, there was proven consanguinity between parents. The geographical origin was: France 6 cases, French Basques 2, Algeria 3, Italy 2, Portugal 2, Tunisia 1, Belgium 1, Switzerland 1, and Argentina 1 case. All patients had been previously treated with androgens and corticosteroids; all except two had been multiply transfused and nine patients were refractory to random platelet transfusions. One patient had multiple liver adenomas which had bled into the peritoneal cavity; these resolved spontaneously after transplantation. All patients had typical cytogenetic abnormalities increased by incubation with nitrogen mustard. They were transplanted from healthy leukocyte antigen (HLA)-identical siblings. All donors were studied for the absence of congenital malformations, the normality of blood counts and the absence of chromosomal breaks on cytogenetic analysis. The patients received a mean cell dose of 4.9×10^8 nucleated cells/kg (range $2.3–9.8 \times 10^8$/kg). The conditioning regimen was well tolerated except in the first five patients who, 2 months after transplantation, developed severe oesophagitis with strictures in three cases. Subsequently, all patients received preventive treatment with ranitidine. This complication is quite unusual after bone marrow transplantation and it is postulated that FA patients may have oesophageal abnormalities which become apparent after irradiation. None of the patients had haemorrhagic cystitis or any other signs of intolerance observed after high-dose cyclophosphamide.

Overall results

Results are shown in Table 3 and Figure 1. Currently 14/19 patients are alive (74%) with a median follow-up time of 4 years (range 6 months to 6 years). Nine patients are doing well without symptoms and with normal development. One patient (SLA 92) had avascular necrosis of the femoral head 2 years after bone marrow transplantation; this was successfully repaired surgically. She developed chronic hepatitis 5 years after bone marrow

Table 3. Bone marrow transplantation results after conditioning with cyclophosphamide 20 mg/kg and 5 Gy thoracoabdominal irradiation.

Patient	Age/sex	Take	A GvHD	C GvHD	Follow-up	Cause of death
SLA 87	15/M	Mixed	0	0	>6 years A/W	
SLA 92	10/F	+	III	0	>5 years A/W	
SLA 97	15/M	Mixed	0	Mild	>5 years A/W	
SLA 100	10/M	+	I	Mild	>5 years A/W	
SLA 101	13/M	+	III	Mild	†996 days	Liver failure + sepsis
SLA 103	12/M	+	II	0	5 years A/W	
SLA 116	5/F	+	II	0	>4 years	
SLA 118	14/M	+	III	NE	†60 days	HUS
SLA 126	17/F	+	III	NE	†104 days	Cmv IP + GvHD
SLA 134	11/F	0	NE	NE	†40 days	*Candida* sepsis
SLA 139	19/M	+	0	0	>3 years A/W	
SLA 141	11/M	+	II	Mild	>3 years A/W	
SLA 148	9/M	+	II	0	>2 years A/W	
SLA 165	12/M	+	II	0	>2 years A/W	
SLA 166	7/M	+	II	0	>2 years A/W	
SLA 180	6/M	Mixed	0	0	>1 year	
SLA 184	12/F	+	I	Mild	>10 months	
SLA 187	20/F	+	III	NE	†58 days GvHD	Aspergillosis
SLA 188	8/M	+	0	0	>6 months	

A GvHD = acute graft versus host disease; C GvHD = chronic graft versus host disease; NE = non-evaluable; A/W = alive and well; HUS = haemolytic and uraemic syndrome; † = died; Cmv IP = cytomegalovirus interstitial pneumonitis.

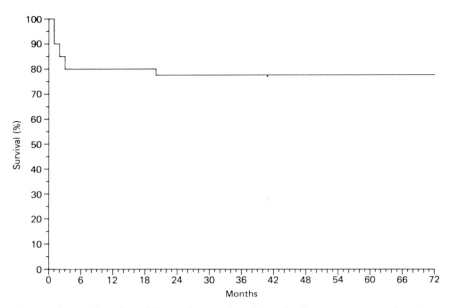

Figure 1. Actuarial survival of Fanconi's anaemia patients after bone marrow transplantation.

transplant which is currently under investigation. Patient SLA 116 was found to be seropositive for human immunodeficiency virus infection; she has subnormal immunological functions and no opportunistic infection. Patient SLA 148 has focal epilepsy related to sequelae of herpes encephalitis which occurred 2 months after transplant. None of the patients developed long-term complications related to the disease or to the conditioning. Secondary malignancies were not observed.

Engraftment

One patient failed to engraft and died on day 40 of *Candida* sepsis. This patient was strongly immunized and severely infected before bone marrow transplant. All the other patients had a prompt take with a mean time to reach $0.5 \times 10^9/l$ granulocytes of 15 days and a mean time to be self-sustaining for platelets of 25 days. One patient, SLA 150, had a take, followed 2 months later by bone marrow failure; cytogenetic analysis showed the existence of a mixed chimerism with a large population of normal lymphocytes without chromosomal breaks and a small population of lymphocytes with the typical abnormalities of FA. His blood counts began to normalize spontaneously 6 months after transplant; 1 year after transplant this patient is doing well, transfusion-free, with mild cytopenia. His cytogenetic analysis shows the persistence of the double population of lymphocytes. This finding prompted us to study the chimerism of our long-term survivors by DNA fingerprinting. So far, three patients have been analysed and despite complete normalization of blood counts, two seem to be mixed chimeras. This represents a striking difference from patients grafted for severe aplastic anaemia where full engraftment has been documented for all the 21 cases of long-term survivors studied (Keable et al, 1987).

From this preliminary analysis we can postulate that the modified conditioning regimen may not be sufficient to allow the establishment of complete chimerism in all cases. This must be studied further.

Graft versus host disease (GvHD)

Acute GvHD, grade II or more, was observed in 11/19 cases (58%). It was treated in the first instance with corticosteroids or, in case of failure, with antilymphocyte-globulin or monoclonal anti-T antibodies (OKT3 or anti-CD8). Eight patients responded; one died on day 996, after bone marrow transplant, of acute liver failure and sepsis. Chronic GvHD was observed in only five cases and was usually limited. Three patients died of acute GvHD; one had an associated haemolytic uraemic syndrome with disseminated intravascular coagulation; one had cytomegalovirus interstitial pneumonitis and one had disseminated aspergillosis.

DISCUSSION

The overall results and complications of this series of patients do not vary markedly from those observed in patients transplanted for other causes of aplastic anaemia. The only difference is the relatively low number of severe chronic GvHD, which is observed in 20% of patients with severe aplastic anaemia. This difference could be due to the small number of patients or perhaps to a defect of FA fibroblasts in producing fibrosis through activation by donor lymphocytes or to the occurrence of a mixed chimerism.

Current results of bone marrow transplantation for non-Fanconi aplastic anaemia have recently been improving, following the same tendency as the FA results: a long-term survival rate of 70% has been obtained by different centres (Hows et al, 1981; Storb et al, 1982; Ramsay et al, 1983; Gluckman et al, 1984a). Several advances have been made in the last decade which explain these results. These include better patient selection, improvement of gnotobiotic care techniques and transfusion support, utilization of new conditioning regimens and immunosuppressive agents such as cyclosporin. A better knowledge of the mechanism of the underlying diseases for which bone marrow transplantation is performed may improve these results further. FA is a good example: it was first shown that patients experienced an unusual toxicity to the conditioning regimen, confirmed by in vitro studies.

Overall, the literature reports a total of 21 patients with FA conditioned with high-dose cyclophosphamide; 38% became long-term survivors with 71% with acute GvHD (Deeg et al, 1983). This result should be compared with that obtained with a modified conditioning regimen which includes no or a very low dose of cyclophosphamide. Besides our own results, Auerbach

showed that FA cells were not more sensitive than normal cells to pro-
carbazine-induced chromosomal breakage (Auerbach, 1981). According to
these results, a conditioning using procarbazine 12.5 mg/kg/day administered in three doses over 6 days, alternating with three doses of antithymocyte globulin (15 mg/kg/day) and followed by low-dose fractionated
total body irradiation (7 Gy) has been used in three patients. This regimen
was well tolerated with mild mucositis. One patient died early of cerebral
haemorrhage, two patients were still alive, but the follow-up was short at the
time of publication.

Subsequently, the decrease or omission of cyclophosphamide from the
conditioning regimen improved the results from 38 to 70% long-term survival rate. Seventeen patients were reported by Hows et al (1987). These
authors used a conditioning regimen similar to the one described above. In
the HLA-identical sibling bone marrow transplantation, survival was 65%.
Patients with non-HLA-identical sibling bone marrow transplantation had a
poor survival (33%); these results are also found in other groups of patients.

Accurate diagnosis of the disease is mandatory. FA is quite different from
the other constitutional aplastic anaemias. Dyskeratosis congenita is clearly
distinguished by its later onset, the occurrence of nail dystrophy and leuko-
plasia of mucosal surfaces and the high frequency of malignant epithelial
tumours. Chromosomal findings have been normal in most published cases
but some authors have described an increased number of chromosomal
breaks. Our own experience clearly separates these two diseases. We had
the opportunity to transplant two patients with dyskeratosis congenita
complicated by severe aplastic anaemia. None had chromosomal abnormalities. They were both conditioned with our severe aplastic anaemia
protocol, including 150 mg/kg cyclophosphamide and 6 Gy thoracoabdominal irradiation. There was no sign of intolerance to cyclophosphamide and the immediate outcome after transplantation was
uneventful. Both developed signs of endothelial activation with diffuse
vasculitis 2 and 7 years after transplantation. These observations suggest
that endothelial cells of dyskeratosis congenita patients may be abnormally
sensitive to the agents used for conditioning.

Accurate diagnosis when familial history is negative or when malformations are not observed is critical. It seems, in the bone marrow transplantation setting, that it is mandatory to test all juvenile aplastic anaemia
patients not only for spontaneous breaks but also for increased breaks after
incubation with appropriate drugs. The standardization of such techniques
would be very useful for the detection of such cases. In our series of 183
patients transplanted for severe aplastic anaemia, the diagnosis of FA was
usually easy. Nevertheless, mistakes were made in two cases. One patient
developed aplastic anaemia at the age of 10 years. He had no malformation
suggestive of FA and no family history. Several cytogenetic studies were
performed; some were normal and one showed 4% chromosomal breakage
with an increase to 16% after incubation with nitrogen mustard. This
abnormality was felt to be insufficient to confirm the diagnosis of FA. The
patient was transplanted at the age of 16 years with cyclophosphamide
150 mg/kg and 6 Gy thoracoabdominal irradiation. Shortly after transplan-

tation, he developed haemorrhagic cystitis, gastrointestinal haemorrhage and skin rash—all symptoms similar to those seen in our first five FA patients transplanted after high-dose cyclophosphamide. He died on day 40 of acute pulmonary oedema. A posteriori, the patient was classified as having FA.

The other patient was diagnosed at 3 months of age with Blackfan–Diamond erythroblastopenia. She had several malformations, including micro-ophthalmia, thumb and skeleton abnormalities, and cardiac malformations similar to those observed in FA. When she was 2 years old, in addition to anaemia, she developed agranulocytosis with repeated severe infectious complications. Her platelet counts remained normal. Repeated cytogenetic analyses were discordant; one showed an increase in chromosomal breaks in peripheral blood lymphocytes while two other analyses were normal without testing the sensitivity to alkylating agents. A study of bone marrow cells showed an increase in chromosomal breaks. Skin tests for radiosensitivity were abnormal. She was conditioned as an FA patient. She had a good take but 6 months after transplantation, she rejected the graft with a reappearance of erythroblastopenia and agranulocytosis.

In conclusion, FA seems to be a potentially curable disease. Prevention could be performed by prenatal diagnosis if there is a positive family history (Auerbach, 1981). Bone marrow transplantation offers a good chance of cure, providing that there is an HLA-identical healthy donor. The chances of finding a donor in FA are slightly higher than usual because of the increased frequency of consanguinity in FA. For those who have no HLA-identical donor, studies are in progress for the use of HLA-matched unrelated donors or for the use of partially mismatched related donors.

REFERENCES

Auerbach AD, Adler B, O'Reilly RJ et al (1983) Effects of procarbazine and cyclophosphamide on chromosome breakage in Fanconi anaemia cells—relevance to bone marrow transplantation. *Cancer Genetics and Cytogenetics* **9**: 25–36.

Beard MEJ (1976) Fanconi anaemia. In *Congenital Disorders of Erythropoiesis*, pp 103–114. Amsterdam: Elsevier Medica North Holland.

Berger R, Bernheim A, Gluckman E et al (1980a) In vitro effect of cyclophosphamide metabolites on chromosomes of Fanconi anaemia patients. *British Journal of Haematology* **45**: 557–564.

Berger R, Bernheim A, Leconiat M et al (1980b) Bone marrow graft of Fanconi's anaemia patient: cytogenetic study. *Cancer Genetics and Cytogenetics* **2**: 127–130.

Deeg HJ, Storb R, Thomas ED et al (1983) Fanconi's anaemia treated by allogeneic bone marrow transplantation. *Blood* **61**: 954–959.

Dutreix J, Wambersie A & Bounik C (1973) Cellular recovery in human skin reactions—application to dose fraction number overall time relationship in radiotherapy. *European Journal of Cancer* **9**: 159–167.

Fanconi G (1967) Familial constitutional panmyelocytopathy Fanconi's anaemia. Clinical aspects. *Seminars in Hematology* **4**: 233–240.

Gluckman E, Devergie A, Schaison G et al (1980) Bone marrow transplantation in Fanconi anaemia. *British Journal of Haematology* **45**: 557–564.

Gluckman E, Devergie A & Dutreix J (1983) Radiosensitivity in Fanconi anaemia, application to the conditioning regimen for bone marrow transplantation? *British Journal of Haematology* **54**: 431–440.

Gluckman E, Devergie A, Benbunan M et al (1984a) Bone marrow transplantation in severe aplastic anaemia using cyclophosphamide and thoraco-abdominal irradiation. In *Aplastic Anaemia—Stem Cell Biology and Advances in Treatment*, pp 325–333. New York: Alan R Liss.

Gluckman E, Devergie A, Poirier O et al (1984b) Use of cyclosporin A as prophylaxis of graft versus host disease after human allogeneic bone marrow transplantation. Report of 38 patients. *Transplantation Proceedings* 15: 2628–2633.

Higurashi M & Conen PE (1971) In vitro chromosomal radiosensitivity in Fanconi's anaemia. *Blood* 38: 336–342.

Hows J, Harris R, Palmer S et al (1981) Immunosuppression with cyclosporin A in allogeneic bone marrow transplantation for severe aplastic anaemia: preliminary results. *British Journal of Haematology* 48: 227–236.

Hows J, Durrant S, Swirkey D, Yin J, Worsley A & Gordon-Smith E (1987) Fanconi's anaemia treated by allogeneic marrow transplantation. *Experimental Hematology* 15: 566.

Keable H, Bourhis JH et al (1987) DNA fingerprinting to study long term chimerism in bone marrow transplantation (BMT) recipients for severe aplastic anaemia (SAA). *Experimental Hematology* 15: 535.

Prindull G, Jentsch E & Hansmann L (1979) Fanconi's anaemia developing erythroleukaemia. *Scandinavian Journal of Haematology* 23: 59–63.

Ramsay NKC, Kim TH, McGlave PB et al (1983) Bone marrow transplantation for severe aplastic anaemia using the conditioning regimen of cyclophosphamide and total lymphoid irradiation. *Experimental Hematology* 10: 139–142.

Storb R, Doney KC, Thomas ED et al (1982) Marrow transplantation with or without donor buffy coat cells for 65 transfused aplastic anaemia patients. *Blood* 59: 236–246.

Swift MR (1976) Fanconi's anaemia: cellular abnormalities and clinical predisposition to malignant disease. In *Congenital Disorders of Erythropoiesis*, pp 11–115. Amsterdam: Elsevier Medica North Holland.

10

Congenital defects of the marrow stem cell

DAVID I. K. EVANS

A variety of rare congenital blood disorders are due to a defect of the bone marrow stem cell. Some, such as Fanconi's anaemia, are due to a profound abnormality of the early non-committed stem cell, and lead to pancytopenia. They are dealt with elsewhere in this volume. This chapter covers the monocytopenias, in which the stem cell abnormality is thought to lie with the committed stem cell. The relationship between these two types is however not always distinct, and some congenital monocytopenias develop into pancytopenia; a terminal transformation to acute leukaemia has been reported in most of these disorders.

In some cases, the evidence for a stem cell defect has not been proved, but such an aetiology seems likely. In others, definite proof exists; the disease has been successfully cured by bone marrow transplantation, both in man and in animals.

DEFECTS OF ERYTHROPOIESIS

Diamond–Blackfan anaemia

Clinical findings

This anaemia was first described from Boston in 1938 as congenital hypoplastic anaemia (Diamond and Blackfan, 1938; Diamond et al, 1976). A total of 25% of cases are anaemic at birth, 65% are anaemic by 6 months, and 90% are anaemic at 1 year. Two thirds of patients show no other defect, but there are two small groups with distinct abnormalities; one group has duplicated, bifid or triphalangeal thumbs and the other group has short webbed necks. Of these cases, some may have other defects, including abnormal facies, snub nose, lip and palate defects, epicanthic folds, hypertelorism, kidney defects, congenital heart disease, mental retardation, hypogonadism, and abnormal eyes (Alter et al, 1981). Clinical signs are summarized in Table 1.

Genetics and aetiology

The inheritance is not clear. There is an increased incidence of birth complications, raising the possibility that some cases are not constitutional but

Table 1. Clinical signs in Diamond–Blackfan syndrome.

Triphalangeal thumbs
Low birthweight and short stature
Abnormal facies
    Snub nose
    Thick upper lip
    Epicanthic folds
    Hypertelorism
Palate and jaw abnormalities
    Cleft palate and/or lip
    Pierre Robin syndrome
    Small jaw
Abnormal ears
Short or webbed neck
Large or small head
Renal abnormalities
Congenital heart disease
Mental retardation
Hypogonadism

Reprinted with permission from Hinchcliffe and Lilley-man, 1987.

rather acquired as a result of complications during delivery. Attempts have been made to demonstrate inhibitors of erythropoiesis, as immune mechanisms have been demonstrated in acquired anaemias due to erythroid hypoplasia. Claims have been made both for (Steinberg et al, 1979) and against (Freedman and Saunders, 1978; Nathan et al, 1978) the presence of T-cell inhibitors of erythropoiesis. Ershler et al (1980) have reported a defect in the bone marrow microenvironment, with good growth of erythroid colonies in vitro. This suggests that the defect lies not with the haemopoietic stem cell but elsewhere.

Nevertheless there is a clear genetic basis. Some cases have shown an autosomal recessive pattern of inheritance. Three fathers have had affected children by different mothers. Cases have also been described in which a parent has shown minor red cell changes without anaemia, such as a modest macrocytosis or increase of fetal haemoglobin (best demonstrated with the Kleihauer test), suggesting a partially expressed form of the disease, passed on in an autosomal dominant manner. There may be several different aetiologies for a disorder which presents with the final picture of erythroid hypoplasia, with different patterns of inheritance and variable associated defects of physical development and bone marrow function. As with other bone marrow diseases, there is a risk of malignancy, and at least three cases have terminated with acute leukaemia.

The association in a child of congenital red cell aplasia, persistent azygous vein continuation of the inferior vena cava, and abnormalities of the forearms, including absent thumbs and hypoplastic radii, was attributed to maternal ingestion of goats' milk contaminated with anagyrine (Ortega and Lazerson, 1987). This suggests that some congenital red cell aplasias may be secondary to toxic effects in utero. Anagyrine is a quinolizidine alkaloid present in plants of the *Lupinus* genus in America. It is known to cause limb abnormalities in the calves of cows who have eaten it during pregnancy; this syndrome is known as crooked calf disease. The calves have bent forelimbs and other abnormalities. This combination of red cell aplasia with a disorder of the preaxial forearm bones is similar to the group of children with red cell aplasia, triphalangeal thumbs, hypoplastic thenar eminences and other abnormalities, first described by Aase and Smith (1969).

Haematological findings

The blood shows anaemia associated with a macrocytosis, with a mean corpuscular volume (MCV) between 100 and 120 fl. Large red cells are a normal finding in the neonate, but in babies affected with Diamond–Blackfan anaemia the MCV remains high as the baby gets older. Some other features of fetal erythropoiesis may be detected, such as a persistence of fetal haemoglobin and the i antigen. The reticulocyte count is low. In some cases the platelet count may be raised and counts of over $1000 \times 10^9/l$ may be found. Platelet function is normal. A few patients have shown neutropenia. Chromosome analysis is normal.

The bone marrow shows a deficiency of normoblasts. This may not always be apparent, as aspiration may by chance draw from an unrepresentative area where there is an erythroid island. In some cases, erythropoiesis may only be depressed and not absent. It should be remembered that the normal response to anaemia is an increase in erythropoiesis, so when an infant is found to be anaemic from most causes, the bone marrow will show increased erythropoiesis. Some authors have commented on an increase in lymphocytes in the bone marrow, raising the possibility that an immune mechanism may be at work. However, the bone marrow of small children normally shows a lymphocyte count as high as 50% in the first months of life, so it is difficult to attribute any significance to this finding. In the neonatal period there is normally also a temporary phase of erythroid depression in the bone marrow, but this does not lead to anaemia. At other times, normoblasts will be found but may show dyserythropoiesis. Finally, it should be remembered that blood transfusion may not only correct anaemia, but also lead to a temporary depression of erythropoiesis, which may lead to confusion with this disease.

One patient showed haematological recovery after bone marrow transplantation (August et al, 1976) but died of post-graft complications on day 55. This suggests a stem cell defect, although the possibility that replacement of the lymphoid system led to endogenous erythroid recovery was not excluded. Four patients were successfully transplanted (Lenarsky et al, 1988).

Metabolic abnormalities

Biochemical defects were at one time thought to be intrinsic to Diamond–Blackfan anaemia. Some patients showed an increased urinary excretion of anthranilic acid, suggesting a defect of tryptophan metabolism, but it is not now believed that this finding is of any importance. A defect of the transport of riboflavin into red cells was described by Mentzer et al (1975). More recently it has been shown that some patients have raised levels of red cell adenosine deaminase (Glader et al, 1983; Whitehouse et al, 1984). Although the finding is not present in any other childhood anaemia, it is again not present in every case. The serum level is high, reflecting poor utilization.

Acquired red cell aplasia

The differential diagnosis of Diamond–Blackfan anaemia includes transient erythroblastopenia of childhood and the acquired aplasia seen in haemolytic anaemias. The main distinguishing feature is that neither of these shows the macrocytosis found in Diamond–Blackfan anaemia. Table 2 compares the three disorders. Transient erythroblastopenia is a disease of toddlers and young children. There may be a preceding history of infection or immunization, but infection of some sort is such a common finding at this age that it is difficult to tell if it plays any part in causing the disease. There is no increase of fetal haemoglobin at diagnosis, although a slight increase may be detected after recovery due to stress erythropoiesis. The disease is self-limiting, but when the anaemia is severe enough to demand treatment, patients respond to corticosteroids or blood transfusion. Temporary depression of erythropoiesis occurs with parvovirus infection, which is normally the cause of erythema infectiosum (fifth disease). When the red cell survival is short, as happens in haemolytic anaemias, a short-lived depression of erythropoiesis causes a marked exacerbation of anaemia.

Other causes of erythroblastopenia include renal failure, which must be excluded in small children with hypoplastic anaemia as the clinical signs of renal disease other than pallor and fatigue may not immediately be apparent. Other causes include vitamin B_2 deficiency, malnutrition and

Table 2. Comparison of three types of erythroblastopenia.

	Diamond–Blackfan syndrome	Transient erythro-blastopenia of childhood	Acute aplastic episode in chronic haemolytic anaemia
Onset	early childhood	usually 1–3½ years	any age
Jaundice	+	+	+
Splenomegaly	0	0	possible
Anaemia	+	+	+
Reticulocytopenia	+	+	+
Neutrophils	N	N	may be low
Platelets	high 80%	N	may be low
MCV	high	N	*
Red cell morphology	macrocytosis	N	*
HbF	raised	N	*
Aetiology	congenital	acquired	acquired (?parvovirus)

MCV = mean corpuscular volume; HbF = haemoglobin F.
* MCV, red cell morphology and haemoglobin F levels will vary depending on the cause of the underlying haemolytic anaemia.
Reprinted with permission from Hinchcliffe and Lilleyman, 1987.

kwashiorkor, the erythroid depression associated with generalized bone marrow failure, leukaemia and lymphoma and osteopetrosis. Drugs and toxins may also depress erythropoiesis. Such drugs include some sedatives, anticonvulsants, antidiabetic agents and heparin. Chloramphenicol produces not only aplastic anaemia, which is an idiosyncratic reaction and may be due to a specific metabolic defect, but also a dose-related depression of erythropoiesis which is non-specific and reversible, and is associated with reticulocytopenia and vacuolation of normoblasts. In adults, erythroblastopenia is commonly acquired and due to immune mechanisms. In 50% of cases there is an associated thymoma. Patients respond to corticosteroids and immunosuppressive drugs.

Treatment

The anaemia in most cases is severe enough to demand treatment. Some babies at diagnosis need blood transfusion, but the mainstay of treatment is corticosteroid therapy, usually given as prednisone or prednisolone. It is important to give a high dose at first, in order to achieve a response. A dose of 20–30 mg prednisone for an infant was recommend by Diamond et al (1976), and an early start to treatment was thought to give a better response. A reticulocytosis usually follows within a week, peaking at 7–10 days. Once a response has been obtained, the dose should be reduced gradually to a maintenance level. It is preferable to aim at a haemoglobin level around 10–11 g/dl with a lower dose of steroid rather than at a normal haemoglobin level with a higher dose. These patients may show reduced stature and it is important to minimize the side-effects of steroids, which are best given on alternate days as is usual with chronic corticosteroid therapy in childhood. Changes are slow to occur. It should be remembered that the drug is acting on the erythroid precursors in the bone marrow, and that the red cells they produce have a normal or near normal survival. It may take several weeks for a change in the steroid dose to be reflected in a change in the haemoglobin level. Three quarters of patients respond to corticosteroids. They may be extremely sensitive to small changes in dosage, so changes should be made slowly. For some patients the clinical severity fluctuates spontaneously. Some patients may recover enough for corticosteroids to be withdrawn temporarily or permanently. Spontaneous remission may rarely occur.

For those patients who do not respond to corticosteroids it is necessary to give regular blood transfusions. This entails all the problems seen with the treatment of thalassaemia major, such as iron overload and antibody formation, and the patients should be managed in a similar way. The author has not found treatment with androgens or vitamin B_6 helpful in such cases, but Diamond et al (1976) found androgens of help in a small number. It is probably worthwhile seeing if a late response to corticosteroids may occur every 3–5 years. It has been reported that high-dose intravenous methylprednisolone (Ozsoylu, 1984) or cyclosporin (Tötterman et al, 1984) may be effective.

Congenital dyserythropoietic anaemia

Various congenital anaemias with ineffective erythropoiesis were classified as congenital dyserythropoietic anaemia types I, II and III by Heimpel and Wendt (1968). Subsequently, cases which did not meet their full criteria were classified as type IV. The patients present with features of a chronic haemolytic anaemia with jaundice, and less frequently with splenomegaly and hepatomegaly. Most cases have been detected in childhood, but some have not been diagnosed until adult life, as the diagnostic features may not be recognized by simple blood tests. The clinical severity is variable, and severe cases may resemble thalassaemia major. The jaundice is due to an unconjugated hyperbilirubinaemia, and fluctuates in its severity. Intercurrent infection may lead to an exacerbation of jaundice and anaemia. The blood film shows macrocytosis, anisocytosis, poikilocytosis and a variety of crenated and contracted cells. There is increased breakdown of red cells and normoblasts, and the damaged cells are removed from the circulation by the reticuloendothelial system, particularly in the spleen. Ferrokinetic studies show ineffective erythropoiesis; an increased amount of iron passes through the plasma, but a decreased amount is incorporated into the red cells. Plasma iron turnover may be increased ten-fold. The red cells may be macrocytic or normocytic, depending on the type, but all show anisocytosis and poikilocytosis. The reticulocyte count is low, which is a feature that indicates a need for bone marrow examination. Cellularity is increased, due to increased erythropoiesis, and there are diagnostic features in the normoblasts, which are of abnormal appearance, sometimes very large, showing megaloblastic features, internuclear chromatin bridges, and double and multiple nuclei. The different types of congenital dyserythropoietic anaemia are shown in Table 3. Although iron overload is a problem, sideroblasts are not a feature of these disorders, with the very rare exception of an unusual variant.

Table 3. Classification of congenital dyserythropoietic anaemia.

Feature	Type I	Type II	Type III
Inheritance	recessive	recessive	dominant
Red cells	macrocytic	normocytic	macrocytic
Normoblast morphology			
Multinuclearity	slight 1–2% binucleated	moderate 20–30% binucleated	prominent gigantoblasts up to 12 nuclei
Megaloblastoid features	yes	no	yes
Internuclear bridges	yes	yes	—
Other features	—	karyorrhexis	—
Serology			
Ham's acid serum test	negative	positive	negative
Sugar water test	negative	negative	negative
Agglutination/haemolysis			
anti-i	negative	+++	weak
anti-I	positive	+++	weak

N.B. Type IV resembles type II with negative acid serum test.

Type I shows macrocytosis, with megaloblastic features in the normoblasts, and internuclear chromatin bridges. Early and intermediate normoblasts are particularly affected. Binuclearity is not prominent (Figure 1a).
Type II shows prominent binuclearity, particularly of the late normoblasts,
multinuclearity and bipolar mitoses, with karyorrhexis (Figure 1b). Type III
shows macrocytosis, with multinuclearity of normoblasts showing as many
as 12 nuclei per cell, and gigantoblasts (Figure 1c).

Similar morphological changes have been recognized in a variety of
acquired disorders. They are not solely limited to congenital disease, but the
serological abnormalities appear to be specific.

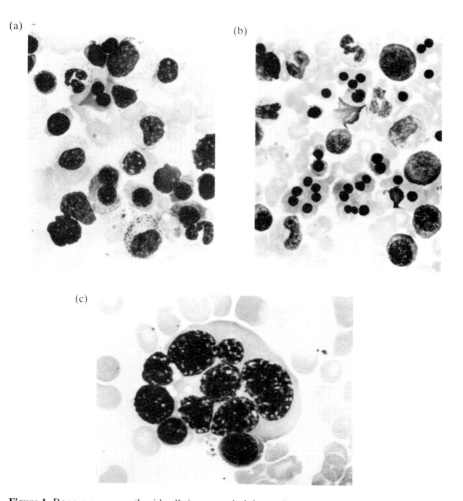

Figure 1. Bone marrow erythroid cells in congenital dyserythropoietic anaemia. **(a)** type I; **(b)**
type II; **(c)** type III.
(by courtesy of Dr SM Lewis and Wm Heinemann Co).

Congenital dyserythropoietic anaemia type I

This variety is rare. Two cases have occurred in families with consanguinity and it seems likely that the disease is usually inherited in an autosomal recessive manner. The heterozygotes cannot be recognized. However, in one family, three sisters and the son of one were affected (Durie et al, 1976), suggesting a dominant inheritance. In another report, the patient's mother showed increased agglutination with anti-i (Castro et al, 1974), suggesting a dominant inheritance with variable expression. There is a chronic refractory macrocytic anaemia with ovalocytosis, teardrop cells and marked aniso-cytosis. The acidified serum test is negative. Positive and negative results have been reported after agglutination with anti-i, and haemolysis with anti-I and complement may be increased or normal. Electron microscopy shows increased folding of the nuclear membrane and loss of the nuclear envelope, chromatin with a spongy appearance, and leakage of chromatin into the cytoplasm.

One case presented with neonatal hyperbilirubinaemia requiring two exchange transfusions (Castro et al, 1974). However, most patients have not been recognized until after the first ten years of life—some not even until over the age of 50. Haemoglobin levels range between 8 and 12 g/dl with reticulocyte counts between 1 and 5%. The anaemia is clearly compatible with normal survival, but with increasing age there is a high risk of gallstones and iron overload with haemosiderosis. The patients show slight jaundice and splenomegaly. A few have also shown skin pigmentation, membranous syndactyly and abnormal hands (Heimpel, 1977). Within the same family, the severity of the anaemia may vary.

Treatment with haematinics and corticosteroids is ineffective. Patients have rarely needed blood transfusion. Although most cases have a large spleen, splenectomy has not been helpful.

Congenital dyserythropoietic anaemia type II

The commonest type is type II, also known as hereditary erythroblastic multinuclearity with a positive acidified acid serum test (HEMPAS; Verwilghen et al, 1973). Less than one quarter of patients are sufficiently anaemic to need blood transfusions, although some women have been transfused during pregnancy. The disease often causes little disability. 90% of patients are jaundiced. 74% have a large spleen, and some improve after splenectomy; 44% have a large liver; some also have cirrhosis or haemo-siderosis of the liver. One in five has gallstones. A few are mentally retarded, and one case had bilateral cataracts. Secondary bone changes are sometimes seen, as in other chronic haemolytic anaemias. Gaucher cells are sometimes present in the bone marrow. The disease is inherited in an autosomal recessive manner. Minor abnormalities of the red cells have been found in symptomless carriers.

Blood tests show a variable haemoglobin level. The reticulocyte count is normal or only slightly raised. The red cells show anisopoikilocytosis with teardrop cells and basophilic stippling. Some red cells may lyse and appear as ghosts. The striking changes in the bone marrow are accompanied by a positive acid serum test, but the sucrose test is negative. About a third of sera used for the test give a positive result. This is due to the presence on the red cells of a specific antigen to which only a minority of normal sera have the necessary IgM anti-HEMPAS antibody. Lysis does not occur with the patient's own serum. The red cells also agglutinate with anti-i antiserum, and reactions may be stronger than seen with normal neonates' red cells. They are also strongly sensitive to lysis with anti-I and complement. These findings all point to a red cell membrane defect, and electron microscopy of the normoblasts shows an extra linear structure parallel to the inside of the cell membrane. It is thought to affect cell division, leading to the characteristic multinuclearity and changes in serology.

Treatment is difficult. Severe anaemia calls for blood transfusion. The usual haematinics are ineffective. Splenectomy may be helpful, and has reduced the transfusion requirement. Many patients have iron overload, and treatment with iron must be avoided. The management of iron overload, with its risk of haemochromatosis and cirrhosis, is now well established in thalassaemia, and patients with a high serum ferritin may benefit from long-term subcutaneous infusion of desferrioxamine, as for that disease. For those who are not very anaemic, unlike patients with thalassaemia major, regular phlebotomy may be an easier alternative.

Congenital dyserythropoietic anaemia type III

This is the rarest form. Inheritance appears to be autosomal dominant. The acid serum test is negative, and the agglutinations with anti-i and anti-I are normal. The giant multinuclear normoblasts are characteristic.

Clinically, the anaemia is of mild to moderate degree. Jaundice and splenomegaly may be present. There may be secondary bone changes.

Congenital dyserythropoietic anaemia type IV

A few patients have been described who do not fit within types I to III. Those showing the morphological features of type II but not the abnormal serology have been classed as type IV. Other isolated cases have shown ringed sideroblasts (Brien et al, 1985), prominent peripheral erythroblastosis (Bethlenfalvay et al, 1985), cytoplasmic inclusions (Kenny et al, 1978), abnormal folate transport (Howe et al, 1979), and membrane changes in granulocyte and platelet, as well as erythrocyte membranes (Lowenthal et al, 1980).

CONGENITAL NEUTROPENIA

Kostmann's syndrome

Kostmann described a severe genetic agranulocytosis in children of Scandinavian origin (Kostmann, 1956, 1975). There is an autosomal recessive pattern of inheritance. There are no other congenital abnormalities. As might be expected with so severe a neutropenia presenting at birth or in early childhood, the patients suffer from recurrent infection which eventually proves fatal. One case survived to develop acute myeloid leukaemia, but most cases have died before the age of 2 years, and have not survived long enough for this complication to have developed. The infections particularly involve the skin, but the umbilicus, ears, lungs and lymph nodes are also affected. They are usually due to pyogenic staphylococci and *Escherichia coli*, and may respond partially to antibiotics, but septicaemia may supervene. Regular prophylactic antibiotics may be helpful; but there is always the risk of development of resistant strains. Regular dental supervision may help prevent the development of oral sepsis. Bone marrow transplantation appears to be the only curative treatment.

The neutrophil count is less than $0.2 \times 10^9/l$ ($200/\mu l$), and the blood film shows a differential count mainly of small lymphocytes with a variable monocytosis. There may sometimes be an eosinophilia. The bone marrow shows no granulocyte development beyond the promyelocyte/myelocyte stage, but the number of CFUc is normal or increased (Amato et al, 1976), suggesting that the defect lies not so much in the stem cell as within the marrow environment. However, Zucker-Franklin et al (1977) demonstrated with electron microscopy that although the colonies appeared grossly normal in size and number, there were many aberrant cells, and concluded that the neutrophil cell line was, after all, intrinsically defective.

Chronic familial neutropenia

Chronic neutropenia is not uncommon, but the aetiology is not well established. Most cases are acquired (Dale et al, 1979) and congenital disease may be difficult to identify in the absence of a positive family history. However, there is a small group of familial neutropenias which are less severe than Kostmann's syndrome, and in which the pattern of inheritance may be autosomal dominant, autosomal recessive, or sex-linked recessive. The patients tend to suffer from recurrent oral infections and ulceration, and from bronchitis, otitis and boils. Infection is common in small children, but patients appear to have fewer infections as they grow older. The usual upper respiratory tract pathogens are commonly involved.

The neutrophil count may fluctuate in the subnormal range or even rise to normal and higher levels with infection. For this reason, some patients may have fewer symptoms than would be expected from the degree of neutropenia. It should be remembered that the neutrophil count measures the number of cells circulating in the blood, whereas infection is governed by the number of neutrophils in the tissues. Some of these patients are able to mobilize an adequate number of neutrophils to sites of infection, even though the transit pool of granulocytes in the blood stream appears reduced. In addition, the monocytosis which may accompany the neutropenia is a further help.

The neutrophils may grow in bone marrow culture without exogenous colony-stimulating factor (Kawaguchi et al, 1985), producing colonies of normal size and type. In contrast to Kostmann's syndrome, the stem cells may be normal. In patients who also show a monocytopenia, the neutropenia may be secondary to lack of colony-stimulating activity which normal monocytes produce (Chilcote et al, 1983).

Cyclical neutropenia

Although this is a rare disease, it has been known for a long time, as the clinical picture of oral sepsis, malaise and pyrexia occurring at regular intervals with recovery in between episodes is distinctive, and was recognized before the neutropenia was identified. It is reviewed by Price and Dale (1978). The term cyclical neutropenia is frequently used loosely to describe any recurrent neutropenia that should properly be described as intermittent. However, the feature *par excellence* of cyclical neutropenia is that it recurs with a regular periodic cycle that is consistent for each patient, and which on average lasts 21 days. The neutrophil count may fluctuate between normal or low normal levels and markedly subnormal levels, often $0.1 \times 10^9/l$ (100/µl) or less.

The onset of neutropenia is frequently heralded by a sense of malaise, and patients may be able to forecast when the count is beginning to fall. This phase corresponds with a maturation arrest of bone marrow granulocytes which is followed 2 or 3 days later by neutropenia and occurrence of symptoms such as mouth ulcers, sore throat, stomatitis and enlarged neck glands. Rectal and vaginal ulceration may occur. There may be abdominal pain, attributed to gastrointestinal ulceration. Recurrent oral sepsis leads to gum infection and permanent dental problems. The ulcers may heal with scarring, and the cervical lymphadenopathy may become chronic.

Other white cells, red cells and platelets are subject to cyclical variation of proliferation but to a lesser degree (Guerry et al, 1973). The neutropenia may be accompanied by a monocytosis. Although there may be a rise and fall in the subnormal neutrophil count of many patients with chronic neutropenia, it is the profound and periodic nature of the change which distinguishes this disease.

Genetics and aetiology

Serial neutrophil counts of other family members, some of whom were symptom-free (Morley et al, 1967), suggested that the disease is inherited in an autosomal dominant manner, with high penetrance and variable expressivity. The monocytosis which accompanies neutropenia in approximately half the cases may also be genetically determined, as these authors showed that it too was a family characteristic. Some of their patients intermittently showed a chronic neutropenia which failed to cycle. Chromosome analysis is normal. Studies on grey collie dogs showed that the disorder is a stem cell defect, which can be transferred from an affected to a normal dog by bone marrow transplantation (Weiden et al, 1973).

Treatment

Although the disease may become less severe with age, 15 deaths were reported by 1981 (Lange and Jones, 1981). No specific treatment has been of great help. A few patients appear to have benefited from androgens or corticosteroids; but in most there is no response and the use of corticosteroids in patients with neutropenia carries the risk of increasing susceptibility to infection. The patient described by Wright et al (1978) who responded to prednisolone was 70 years old, suggesting that the disease was of a milder type than usual, or not genetic in origin. Lithium merely amplified the granulocyte oscillation in the patient of von Schulthess et al (1983), but she improved after a course of plasmapheresis and become asymptomatic. One of the author's patients showed a temporary response to an infusion of plasma (Evans and Holzel, 1968). Splenectomy has resulted in higher neutrophil counts, but with the continuation of cycling.

Infective episodes demand treatment with antibiotics. Unless the infection can be cured before the next drop of the neutrophil count, there is a danger that the infection will become chronic. It may be necessary to continue antibiotics for several cycles. One of the author's patients is helped by a short course of co-trimoxazole, taken at the onset of each 3 weekly cycle.

Miscellaneous neutropenias

Congenital dysgranulopoietic neutropenia

A small subgroup of patients with congenital neutropenia may also have dysgranulopoiesis (Parmley et al, 1980). The bone marrow may show multinucleated neutrophil promyelocytes to polymorphs with as many as 4 to 16 nuclei or more nuclear lobes (Lightsey et al, 1985). The neutrophils show cytoplasmic vacuoles, autophagy and lipid inclusions. Primary granules are defective or degenerate. Mature neutrophils are difficult to identify, because of the neutropenia, but secondary granules are absent or decreased. Cytochemistry shows abnormal alkaline phosphatase but normal peroxidase. Electron microscopy demonstrates abnormalities of cytoplasmic maturation. Lactoferrin may be absent. Monocytes, macrophages, lymphocytes and eosinophils are normal. Bone marrow culture shows normal CFU and normal CSF. No serum inhibitors of granulopoiesis are present.

The patients all suffer from serious life-threatening bacterial infections. *Pseudomonas* cellulitis of the perirectal area, groin and face has been described, as well as recurrent lung abscesses with *Pseudomonas*. Other bacteria isolated include *Klebsiella*, *Staphylococcus*, *Escherichia coli*, *Clostridium clostridiiforme* and *Bacteroides*. Two of the six cases described by Parmley et al (1980) died. The neutrophil counts rarely exceeded $0.3 \times 10^9/l$ (300/μl). However, the disease ran a more serious course in children under the age of 2 years. As happens with other chronic neutropenias, the clinical severity moderates with increasing age. The disease was so called because the abnormalities of the neutrophil series recalled those seen in congenital dyserythropoietic anaemia.

This is a severe disease with a poor prognosis. Antibiotic treatment is frequently needed, and the management is the same as for severe neutropenias such as Kostmann's syndrome. The presence of *Pseudomonas* infection is probably the result of treatment with multiple antibiotics rather than of a specific feature of the disease. Parmley et al (1980) treated their cases with leukocyte transfusions. This is not usually justified for recurrent congenital neutropenia, but the fact that the disease appears to be less severe after the age of 2 years might justify an optimistic approach in young children. The severity of the disease justifies bone marrow transplantation.

Myelokathexis

Zuelzer (1964) described a patient with chronic neutropenia whose neutrophils had a bizarre appearance of the nuclei with long thin filaments between the lobes, and which also showed defective mobility and phagocytosis. In another family, the father and daughter were similarly affected, and also had hypogammaglobulinaemia (Mentzer and Johnston, 1977).

Familial neutropenia with immune defect

Several reports have described cases with a familial incidence of neutropenia and a variety of immune deficiencies, including humoral and cellular defects, and combined defects such as the cartilage–hair hypoplasia syndrome. In these cases it seems likely that the neutropenia is secondary and of immune origin, and that it is the immune defect which is hereditary.

Lazy leukocyte syndrome

Two children were described by Miller et al (1971) who presented with the usual symptoms of neutropenia—stomatitis, gingivitis, otitis and pyrexia. The peripheral blood showed a profound neutropenia with neutrophils in the range of 0.1 to 0.2 × 10^9/l (100–200/µl). In contrast to other neutropenias, the number of granulocyte precursors and mature neutrophils in the bone marrow was normal. A defect of chemotaxis and random mobility was demonstrated in vitro, and the neutrophils showed reduced ability to migrate into a skin abrasion in vivo. The neutrophil response to endotoxin was abnormal. Phagocytic and bactericidal activity were normal.

It was postulated that the neutrophils were unable to migrate from the bone marrow to the blood and sites of infection, and so were considered 'lazy'. The neutrophils showed normal morphology, and normal phagocytic and bactericidal activity. The serum produced chemotactic factors normally. Cellular and humoral immune function were normal.

This disease might be suspected when a patient with a significant neutropenia is found to have a normal number of mature and developing granulocytes in the bone marrow. A defect of chemotaxis (provided enough neutrophils can be obtained to test) would be a confirmatory finding. The clinical findings, however, do not distinguish these patients from other cases with severe chronic neutropenia. Management is the same as for other chronic neutropenias.

176   D. I. K. EVANS

Reticular dysgenesis

Less then ten cases of this rare disorder have been described. Patients all die
from a combination of severe combined immune deficiency with agranulocytosis in the first months of life (de Vaal and Seynhaave, 1959). There is a
profound lymphoid deficiency in all tissues; the only immunoglobulin
detected is of maternal origin, and the bone marrow shows a complete
absence of granulocyte precursors, with normal megakaryocytes, normoblasts and reticular tissue. The disease is attributed to a defect of bone
marrow differentiation at the tenth week of fetal development.

Chediak–Higashi syndrome

Patients with the Chediak–Higashi syndrome suffer from frequent and
severe pyogenic infections with staphylococci and streptococci due to
abnormal neutrophil function. There is a generalized lysosomal defect of all
body cells, leading to reduced pigmentation and partial albinism. They have
a greyish sheen to their hair, light skin, retinal albinism with photophobia,
and may develop hepatosplenomegaly, generalized lymphadenopathy, and
terminal lymphohistiocytic malignancy.

The neutrophils contain abnormally large specific granules, 2–4 μ in
diameter (Figure 2). The lymphocytes may contain a single large azurophilic
granule. Leukopenia is frequent, and the abnormality may not be visible in
all the neutrophils. Consequently the abnormality may be difficult to recognize on a superficial examination of the blood film. The changes can be
recognized in the developing cells of the bone marrow, together with vacuolation of the granulocytes and large inclusions in the promyelocytes. The
bone marrow is hypercellular.

The neutrophils show defects of chemotaxis, degranulation and bacterial
killing (Boxer et al, 1976). Peripheral blood lymphocytes and NK-enriched
large granular lymphocytes show negligible activity against several target
cells (Nair et al, 1987).

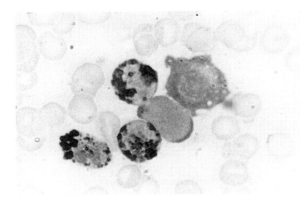

Figure 2. Chediak–Higashi syndrome. Bone marrow granulocytes stained with Sudan black to
show the giant specific granules.

There is also a bleeding disorder due to platelet storage pool deficiency (Apitz-Castro et al, 1985).

Genetics and aetiology

The disorder is well recognized in many other mammals including mink, cattle, foxes, cats and mice. It is inherited in an autosomal recessive manner. The carriers may show an increased antibody response to Epstein–Barr virus capsid antigen, and a defective response to the diffuse component of the early antigen, with low NK cells and increased suppressor cells (Merino et al, 1986).

The inclusions in the cells are giant lysosomes, and are formed by a process of fusion, cytoplasmic injury and phagocytosis (Barak and Nir, 1987). They can also be found in fibroblasts, histiocytes, renal tubular epithelium and neurones. Fibroblasts show a significant reduction of activity of α-D-mannose (Miller et al, 1986). The defect results in delayed delivery of lysosomal contents into phagosomes. Cyclic adenosine monophosphate levels are high. Cyclic guanosine monophosphate improves microtubular function and neutrophil function in patients with the disease (Boxer et al, 1977), and it is thought that there is a defect of microtubular assembly. Ascorbic acid may also affect microtubular function, and improve the defect (Boxer et al, 1976). The defect of lymphocyte function may account for the predisposition to malignant disease.

Patients infected with Epstein–Barr virus showed a prolonged hepato-splenomegaly and lymphadenopathy, with immune responses similarly abnormal to those reported in carriers, suggesting an immunodeficiency to this virus (Merino et al, 1986).

Treatment

Antibiotics are given for infective episodes, which are usually caused by Gram-positive bacteria. The principles of treatment follow those recommended for other neutrophil defects and neutropenias. Prophylactic antibiotics have not proved helpful and are not recommended.

When the malignant phase develops with hepatosplenomegaly and lymphadenopathy due to lymphohistiocytic infiltration, treatment with high doses of corticosteroids, vincristine, antimetabolites and alkylating agents has shown some success (Blume and Wolff, 1972) but there are no more recent reports. One patient in the accelerated phase showed improvement with intravenous gammaglobulin (Kinugawa and Ohtani, 1985). This phase may be more a reactive proliferation than a true malignancy, so treatment of the immunological abnormality is logical.

The use of ascorbic acid, mentioned above, has the benefit of being harmless and simple. As the disease has been cured in animals by bone marrow transplantation, it should be considered for treatment of humans too.

Shwachman syndrome

Clinical features

Shwachman et al (1964) first described this disease which was confused with cystic fibrosis, as the patients presented with recurrent chest infections, diarrhoea and failure to thrive. However, whereas both diseases show defective pancreatic function, only Shwachman's syndrome is associated with a bone marrow disorder. A total of 95% of cases show neutropenia; 70% show thrombocytopenia and 50% are anaemic. The disorder is reviewed by Schmerling et al (1969) and Aggett et al (1980). Unlike cystic fibrosis, there is no generalized defect of exocrine secretion, and levels of sodium and chloride in the sweat are normal.

The patients are usually small. They may have a low birthweight, and neonatal problems are common, affecting 80% of cases. Their skeletal maturation is delayed. They fail to thrive, and the onset of puberty starts late. Young children show bone abnormalities of the ribs, which are abnormally short, with flared ends. Older patients show metaphyseal chondrodysplasia (see Figure 3), most frequently affecting the head of the femur, but also the knee, humeral head, wrist, ankle and vertebra. The long bones may be bowed. The fingers may show clinodactyly.

The exocrine pancreatic deficiency leads to chronic diarrhoea. The degree of pancreatic defect and consequent malabsorption is variable. The pancreas is fatty and hypoplastic or degenerative. In young children, the liver may be enlarged and liver function tests may be abnormal. The defects may correct themselves as the child grows, suggesting that this is a temporary fatty infiltration secondary to malnutrition and infection.

Recurrent infection is a problem, and the frequency of infection appears disproportionate to the degree of neutropenia compared to patients with simple neutropenia, as in aplastic anaemia. There is no specific infectious organism, but like other patients with neutrophil defects, the children develop superficial sepsis with boils, recurrent otitis, gingivitis and pyorrhoea, and upper and lower respiratory tract infection. Other defects reported include Hirschsprung's disease, diabetes mellitus, dental abnormalities, myocardial disease and a variety of other dysplastic features. An ichthyotic maculopapular rash was present in 65% of the cases reported by Aggett et al (1980). Although the original report of Shwachman et al (1964) mentioned normal motor and mental development, hypotonia, developmental delay, abnormal photic sensitivity and a low intelligence quotient have subsequently been described.

Respiratory function tests show a reduced thoracic gas volume and chest wall compliance in small children, and a reduced forced expiratory volume and forced vital capacity in order patients. This feature may be associated with the rib abnormalities, and contributes to chest infections.

A few reports have commented upon the presence of galactosuria, glycosuria, hyperaminoaciduria, and nephrocalcinosis. Renal tubular acidosis has been recognized (Marra et al, 1986), and may be more common than is generally supposed. It may contribute to the failure to thrive.

The clinical findings are summarized in Table 4.

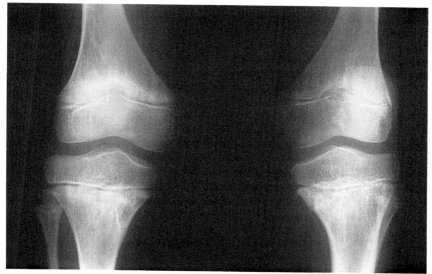

(a)

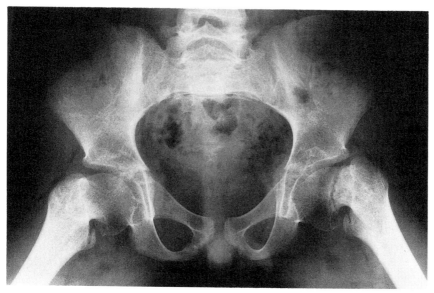

(b)

Figure 3. Metaphyseal dysplasia in Shwachman's syndrome. (a) There are marked metaphyseal changes in the upper ends of both tibiae with irregularity of the epiphyseal plate and abnormal ossification within the metaphysis and patchy sclerosis. The lower femora are both expanded, with notching of the epiphysis. (b) Bilateral coxa vara. There is a fracture through the left femoral neck. (by courtesy of Dr JF Ratcliffe).

Table 4. Features of Shwachman's
syndrome.

Exocrine pancreatic deficiency
Poor growth and delayed puberty
Steatorrhoea and malabsorption
Recurrent infection
Neutropenia
Defective neutrophil chemotaxis
Abnormal lung function
Bone abnormalities
Metaphyseal dyschondroplasia
Delayed bone age
Rib defects
Bone marrow disorder
Neutropenia
Thrombocytopenia
Anaemia
Bone marrow hypoplasia
Bone marrow dysplasia
Neonatal problems
Psychomotor retardation
Hypotonia
Renal tubular defects
Hepatomegaly and abnormal liver function
Dysmorphic features
Diabetes mellitus
Chronic lung disease
Dysgammaglobulinaemia

Genetics and aetiology

This is a genetically determined disease, although the pattern of inheritance
is not completely clear. Multiple cases have occurred in one family. The
pattern of inheritance is likely to be autosomal recessive, with variable
penetrance. No consistent chromosome abnormality has been described.
The cause for Shwachman's syndrome is not known, but Aggett et al (1980)
proposed that it is due to defective function of microtubules and micro-
filament elements, affecting cartilage, neutrophils and pancreatic cells.

Haematological features

The blood may show a variety of disorders including anaemia, neutropenia
and thrombocytopenia, either singly or in combination. However, the most
prominent abnormality is neutropenia, although it may be intermittent. The
neutrophil count is generally less than $1.5 \times 10^9/l$ ($1500/\mu l$). The platelet
count is frequently less than $100 \times 10^9/l$ ($100000/\mu l$). Not only does the bone
marrow show a deficiency of the precursors of mature blood cells, but also a
variety of morphological abnormalities. There may be dyserythropoiesis
and a raised level of fetal haemoglobin, dysgranulopoiesis and abnormal
megakaryocyte morphology (Figure 4a). Such changes are often present in
all the bone marrow cells, even when only one cell line is reduced in number

in the peripheral blood. Nevertheless, there may be enough reserve of granulocytes in the bone marrow and elsewhere for the patient to show a neutrophil leukocytosis with infection. A small number of patients have shown a more profound bone marrow defect, showing a pancytopenia with bone marrow changes of aplastic anaemia. The features in these cases are no different from those found in other aplastic anaemias. Mast cells are often prominent, even in cases without overt aplasia (Figure 4b). At least two cases have developed acute leukaemia.

Aggett et al (1979) described defective neutrophil mobility in the greater majority of the cases they studied. Rothbaum et al (1982) reported a uniquely abnormal surface distribution and mobility of concanavalin A receptors in about a third of neutrophils of the three cases they studied. They concluded that this was evidence for a cytoskeletal defect and that it might contribute to the defect of chemotaxis. It is likely that the explanation for the susceptibility to infection lies not only with the neutropenia, but also with these defects of neutrophil function, together with a contribution from the abnormalities of lung function already mentioned.

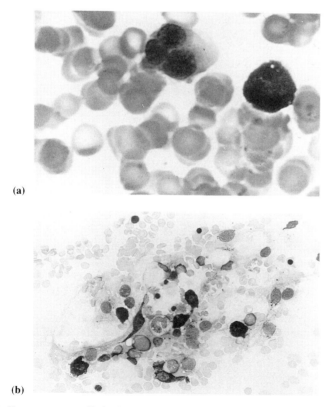

(a)

(b)

Figure 4. Bone marrow cells in Shwachman's syndrome. (a) Trinucleated normoblast. (b) Multiple mast cells in bone marrow smear.

Treatment

Control of diarrhoea and malabsorption are the main problems of management. As with other cases with pancreatic failure, pancreatic extracts are given mixed with food or in divided doses before, during and after meals. The dose is regulated according to the size, number and consistency of the stools, and by the patient's general progress. Extra allowances may be needed if snacks are taken between meals, which may be necessary to increase calorie intake. As some pancreatic preparations are broken down by stomach acids, a dose of cimetidine or ranitidine may be helpful, taken 30–45 minutes before the pancreatic preparation. This reduces stomach acid secretion and potentiates the action of the enzyme.

Increased amounts of dietary proteins and calories may be necessary, and patients should be given regular vitamin supplements. The levels of calcium, magnesium, iron and other minerals should be monitored regularly, and any deficiency corrected appropriately. A gluten-free diet is unlikely to be helpful.

The haematological management is less demanding. A watch should be kept for the development of iron deficiency anaemia, as pancreatic supplements tend to reduce iron absorption. Folic acid deficiency may sometimes develop. If it does, regular folate supplements are justified, but not all patients need them. Severe anaemia will require blood transfusion. If the neutropenia leads to recurrent sepsis, it is sensible to prescribe long-term antibiotic cover; the author has found that prophylactic co-trimoxazole may be helpful, as with other patients with increased susceptibility to infection. Isolated episodes of bacterial infection require cultures to be taken for bacterial isolation and antibiotic-sensitivity tests. The appropriate antibiotics should be given. Because of malabsorption, oral absorption may be uneven and antibiotics given by mouth may be ineffective. It may be necessary to use the parenteral route. Bleeding from thrombocytopenia is not usually severe, and usually presents as an increased tendency to bruise. Haematologists should however remember that vitamin K deficiency may develop with malabsorption, and the coagulation status should be monitored, particularly if there is an exacerbation of bruising. Furthermore, liver disease is a complication of the syndrome, and a prolonged prothrombin time may reflect poor liver function rather than vitamin K deficiency. Regular vitamin K prophylaxis is not usually necessary. Platelet transfusions should be avoided, as with other chronic thrombocytopenias, in order to avoid the development of platelet antibodies, with a consequent failure to respond to random platelet transfusions.

Szüts et al (1984) found that intramuscular administration of thiamine 5 mg/kg daily for 5 days corrected the defect of chemotaxis in two affected boys, with clinical improvement which lasted for 10 weeks. A repeat treatment produced a similar benefit. Regular thiamine supplements may be beneficial.

AMEGAKARYOCYTIC THROMBOCYTOPENIAS

Although this group of disorders are called amegakaryocytic, bone marrow examination shows that the megakaryocytes are not absent, but reduced in number. They are frequently small, immature and dysplastic. In some disorders they may also show defective function. The term is retained to describe several disorders, both congenital and acquired, in which a low platelet count is due to reduced platelet production with normal numbers of erythroid and white cells. In contrast to the acquired thrombocytopenias of immune origin, these disorders respond well to platelet transfusions. Unfortunately random platelet transfusions may lead to the development of antiplatelet antibodies and a failure to respond, so they should be reserved for life-threatening episodes.

Thrombocytopenia-absent radius (TAR) syndrome

Babies with this disease are born with abnormally short forearms and radial deviation of the hand which is hypoplastic. The radial aplasia is always bilateral, and the thumbs are always present. Some babies may develop cerebral haemorrhage during delivery or shortly afterwards. Half the babies develop thrombocytopenia within the first week of life, and 90% are affected by the first 4 months, developing petechiae and melaena. These children are of normal weight at birth, but frequently become small and underweight as they grow older. A small jaw, abnormal shoulders, dislocated hips and club feet can be associated findings. A third have congenital heart disease, and a third have absence of the ulna (Hall et al, 1969). The spleen is sometimes enlarged. If the child survives the first weeks and months of life, the prognosis is good. The disease has been described in both white and black children (Adeyokunnu, 1984).

It should be noted that radial aplasia can also exist as an isolated disorder, sometimes unilaterally. Furthermore, the syndrome is quite distinct from Fanconi's anaemia, although forearm abnormalities are also seen in that disease too. Nor is there any predisposition to malignancy. Some patients with trisomy 18 have forearm abnormalities and thrombocytopenia, but the associated defects are more extensive than found in the TAR syndrome.

Laboratory findings

Platelet counts are usually less than $50 \times 10^9/l$ (50 000/μl) at diagnosis, and are of normal size. The megakaryocytes are small, dysplastic and reduced in number. In the immediate neonatal period, babies may have a high white cell count, up to $100 \times 10^9/l$ (100 000/μl) and rarely higher, due to a granulocytosis, which may be accompanied by the presence of myelocytes and other primitive granulocytes in the blood. This gives the appearance of a leukaemoid reaction. An eosinophilia is common. Apart from reactive changes, the normoblasts and white cells are normal.

The leukocytosis settles within a few months, although occasional myelocytes may be seen in the blood for longer. As the children get older, the purpura often improves, but not as quickly as the leukocytosis. The bleeding time may become normal as the years go by, but although the platelet count may slowly rise, it does not become normal.

A small number of cases have been reported with abnormal platelet function, but no consistent abnormality is present. Some cases have had agammaglobulinaemia.

Genetics and aetiology

The disease is inherited in an autosomal recessive manner, but girls are affected twice as often as boys. Unlike Fanconi's anaemia, there is no chromosome defect. The disease is not due to drug ingestion such as thalidomide.

In some cases there appears to be an allergy to cows' milk, which causes gastrointestinal bleeding, failure to thrive and diarrhoea (Hall et al, 1969; Whitefield and Barr, 1976). It has been shown that cows' milk proteins may combine with IgG antibodies to form immune complexes which may bind to platelets, megakaryocytes and gastrointestinal blood vessels (Delire et al, 1978), causing an exacerbation of bleeding (Stuart and McKenna, 1981).

Treatment

As stated above, platelet transfusions should be reserved for severe bleeding episodes. Irradiated platelets should be considered for cases with severe defect of cellular immunity. There is no response to corticosteroids, androgens or splenectomy. The latter is not advisable in small children because of the risk of postsplenectomy sepsis. In older children, whose platelet count may have improved, operation may be undertaken without platelet support.

The forearm deformity should be treated with splints and massage, in order to minimize the radial deviation which can progress with age. The results of orthopaedic surgery in the author's experience have been disappointing. It should be remembered that the whole forearm is hypoplastic, with weak and absent muscles as well as bone defects. The absence of the radius means that there is no platform for articulation of the wrist. Children are able to write and use their abnormal hands surprisingly well. Fixation of the forearm with the hand straight may improve the appearance of the hand, at the expense of function. Operations to release tight tendon bands may be helpful, but unless incapacitating deformity has been allowed to develop, it is preferable to leave corrective operations for as long as possible.

For those children who show signs of cows' milk allergy or who present with gastrointestinal bleeding a milk-free diet should be recommended.

Wiskott–Aldrich syndrome

Affected patients are male, and thrombocytopenia is associated with eczema and an immune defect. Bleeding may present in the first weeks or months of life, with bloody diarrhoea, bleeding eczema or nappy rash. Incomplete forms of the disease are common (Standen et al, 1986), so purpura may be only slight, eczema may be mild or intermittent, and evidence of immune deficiency may be absent. Some cases described as simple sex-linked thrombocytopenia may be partly expressed forms of Wiskott–Aldrich syndrome. One varient shows high serum IgA and renal disease.

Patients may develop a variety of allergies, including cow's milk allergy, and in this way resemble the cases of TAR syndrome described above. The immune defect may lead to recurrent chest and bowel infections. Recurrent otitis is a problem. Infection is due to a variety of organisms, including bacteria, viruses, fungi and *Pneumocystis carinii*. As with other immune deficiency states, there is a predisposition to malignant disease, which usually presents as a lymphohistiocytic proliferative disorder. Death is usually due to bleeding, infection or malignancy, and only a minority of patients survive after the age of ten.

Laboratory findings

The platelet count is usually less than $50 \times 10^9/l$ ($50\,000/\mu l$). The platelets are small, with an MCV about 5–6 cμ, and a deficiency of dense bodies. Small platelets in any boy with thrombocytopenia should make one suspect the syndrome. Thrombocytopenia is usually attributed to defective mega-karyopoiesis, but autoimmune mechanisms have also been described. A defect of platelet function is sometimes present, corresponding to a storage pool defect. The platelets may be removed from the circulation prematurely by the reticuloendothelial system. Bone marrow megakaryocytes are small and dysplastic. There is frequently an eosinophilia and a lymphopenia. There is no primary defect of red cells or granulocytes.

Immunological findings include T-cell deficiency, which may lead to a low blood lymphocyte count. The lymphocytes respond poorly to mitogens and polysaccharide antigens. There may be dysgammaglobulinaemia, with low IgM. Because blood group substances and pneumococci are polysaccharides, levels of anti-A and anti-B may be absent or low, and there is a defective immune response against pneumococci. Levels of IgE may be very high, and reaginic antibodies may be found.

Histology of the lymph nodes shows reticular hyperplasia, absence of germinal centres, and depletion of the T-cell areas in the paracortical region.

Genetics and aetiology

This is a sex-linked recessive disease. Carrier females are symptom-free and cannot be recognized by normal laboratory investigation. The gene has not been identified yet, but has been localized to the pericentric region of the X chromosome (Peacocke & Simanovitch, 1987). Electron microscopy shows that the lymphocytes lack the microvilli seen on normal lymphocytes (Kenney et al, 1986). They also show a defective form of sialophorin (Remold–O'Donnell et al, 1984). This is a heavily sialated surface protein, previously called gpL115, which is present on normal lymphocytes and platelets, but not on erythrocytes and fibroblasts (Remold–O'Donnell et al,

1987). One family showed loose linkage with the L1 DNA marker (Standen, 1988).

Treatment

Platelet transfusions produce a good increment initially, but should be reserved for life-threatening bleeding. These boys may produce antibodies readily, including antibodies against transfused platelets with failure to respond to unselected platelets. If the patient has a severe defect of cellular immunity, there may be a possibility of graft versus host disease, so platelets and other blood products could with advantage be irradiated.

Corticosteroids and androgens are without benefit on the platelet count. However, corticosteroids may benefit the eczema, with the result that patients so treated, whose eczema disappears, may not be diagnosed. Long-term corticosteroids affect the immune response adversely, and should therefore be used with care in these boys.

Splenectomy may improve the platelet count. Unfortunately, the patients are exceptionally prone to postsplenectomy sepsis with pneumococci. Prophylaxis with pneumococcal vaccines is ineffective, as the patients cannot respond to them. Consequently, penicillin should be given to every splenectomized patient with the Wiskott–Aldrich syndrome for the rest of his life. The operation is not generally advisable for this disease.

Treatment with transfer factor has helped the clinical condition and immune disorder in a few patients. Bone marrow transplantation has cured both the immune defect and the thrombocytopenia, and is the treatment of choice for severely affected boys with a suitable donor.

Patients may develop a variety of dietary allergies, including allergy to cows' milk, eggs and other animal proteins. Affected boys with failure to thrive and diarrhoea should not only be investigated for chronic intestinal infection with giardia, cryptosporidium, bacteria and viruses, but should also be tried on an exclusion diet.

Amegakaryocytic thrombocytopenia

There is a very rare disorder in which isolated thrombocytopenia in the neonatal period is followed by the development of aplastic anaemia. Seven cases were described by O'Gorman-Hughes (1974) with isolated neonatal thrombocytopenia; aplastic anaemia developed several months to 12½ years later. Four cases were described by Alter et al (1981), one of whom died of acute myeloid leukaemia at the age of 16 years, having become aplastic at the age of 2. Other isolated cases have been reported. The patients show no associated physical abnormalities and signs are related solely to the thrombocytopenia. Bone marrow megakaryocytes are scanty or absent and appear dysplastic.

The disease is thought to be congenital, but is distinct from Fanconi's anaemia, although in this disorder thrombocytopenia frequently precedes the development of overt marrow failure too. Chromosome analysis is normal (Saunders and Freedman, 1978). Other cases with amegakaryocytic thrombocytopenia include the family described by Myllyla et al (1967) who had thrombocytopenia with an autosomal recessive pattern of inheritance. Amegakaryocytic thrombocytopenia in the newborn can also occur as a transitory disorder, due to maternal antiplatelet antibodies with human leukocyte antigen specificity (Evans, 1987). Such patients are capable of developing full recovery without bone marrow failure.

REFERENCES

Aase JM & Smith DW (1969) Congenital anaemia and triphalangeal thumbs: a new syndrome. *Journal of Pediatrics* **74**: 471–474.

Adeyokunnu AA (1984) Radial aplasia and amegakaryocytic thrombocytopenia (TAR syndrome) among Nigerian children. *American Journal of Diseases of Children* **138**: 346–348.

Aggett PJ, Harries JT, Harvey BAM & Soothill JF (1979) An inherited defect of neutrophil mobility in Shwachman's syndrome. *Journal of Pediatrics* **94**: 391–394.

Aggett PJ, Cavanagh NPC, Matthew DJ, Pincott JR, Sutcliffe J & Harries JT (1980) Shwachman's syndrome. *Archives of Disease in Childhood* **55**: 331–347.

Alter BP, Rappeport JM & Parkman R (1981) The bone marrow failure syndromes. In Nathan DG & Oski FA (eds) *Hematology of Infancy and Childhood* 2nd edn pp 168–249. Philadelphia: WB Saunders.

Amato D, Freedman MH & Saunders EF (1976) Granulopoiesis in severe congenital neutropenia. *Blood* **47**: 531–538.

Apitz-Castro R, Cruz MR, Ledezma E et al (1985) The storage pool deficiency in platelets from humans with the Chediak–Higashi syndrome: study of six patients. *British Journal of Haematology* **59**: 471–483.

August CS, King E, Githens JH et al (1976) Establishment of erythropoiesis following bone marrow transplantation in a patient with congenital hypoplastic anaemia (Diamond–Blackfan syndrome). *Blood* **48**: 491–498.

Barak Y & Nir E (1987) Chediak–Higashi syndrome. *American Journal of Pediatric Hematology and Oncology* **9**: 42–55.

Bethlenfalvay NC, Hadnagy CS & Heimpel H (1985) Unclassified type of congenital dyserythropoietic anaemia (CDA) with prominent peripheral erythroblastosis. *British Journal of Haematology* **60**: 541–550.

Blume RS & Wolff SM (1972) The Chediak–Higashi syndrome: studies in four patients and a review of the literature. *Medicine* **51**: 247–280.

Boxer LA, Watanabe AM, Rister M, Besch HR, Jr, Allen J & Baehner RL (1976) Correction of leucocyte function in Chediak–Higashi syndrome by ascorbate. *New England Journal of Medicine* **295**: 1041–1045.

Boxer LA, Rister M, Allen JM & Baehner RL (1977) Improvement of Chediak–Higashi leukocyte function by cyclic guanosine monophosphate. *Blood* **49**: 9–17.

Brien WF, Mant MJ & Etches WS (1985) Variant congenital dyserythropoietic anaemia with ringed sideroblasts. *Clinical and Laboratory Haematology* **7**: 231–237.

Castro O, Nash I & Finch SC (1974) Congenital dyserythropoietic anaemia type I. Report of a case with increased erythrocyte agglutinability by anti-i serum. *Archives of Internal Medicine* **134**: 346–351.

Chilcote RR, Rierden WJ & Baehner RL (1983) Neutropenia, recurrent bacterial infections, and congenital deafness in patients with monocytopenia. *American Journal of Diseases of Children* **137**: 964–967.

Dale DC, Guerry DM, Wewerka JR, Bull JM & Chusid MJ (1979) Chronic neutropenia. *Medicine* **58**: 128–144.

Delire M, Cambiaso CL, Masson PL (1978) Circulating immune complexes in infants fed on cow's milk. *Nature* **272**: 632.

de Vaal OM & Seynhaave V (1959) Reticular dysgenesis. *Lancet* **ii**: 1123–1125.

Diamond LK & Blackfan KD (1938) Hypoplastic anemia. *American Journal of Diseases in Childhood* **56**: 464–467.

Diamond LK, Wang WC & Alter BP (1976) Congenital hypoplastic anemia. In Schulman I (ed.) *Advances in Pediatrics*, vol. 22, pp 349–378. Chicago: Year Book Medical Publishers.

Durie BGM, Payne C, Kim HD et al (1976) Detailed studies of unusual membrane abnormalities in a family with congenital dyserythropoietic anaemia type I. *Blood* **48**: 963.

Ershler WB, Ross J, Finlay JL & Shahidi NT (1980) Bone-marrow microenvironment defect in congenital hypoplastic anemia. *New England Journal of Medicine* **302**: 1321–1327.

Evans DIK (1987) Immune amegakaryocytic thrombocytopenia of the newborn: association with anti-HLA-A2. *Journal of Clinical Pathology* **40**: 258–261.

Evans DIK & Holzel A (1968) Cyclical neutropenia. *Proceedings of the Royal Society of Medicine* **61**: 302.

Freedman MH & Saunders EF (1978) Diamond–Blackfan syndrome: evidence against cell-mediated erythropoietic suppression. *Blood* **51**: 1125.

Glader BE, Backer K & Diamond LK (1983) Elevated erythrocyte adenosine deaminase activity in congenital hypoplastic anemia. *New England Journal of Medicine* **309**: 1486–1490.

Guerry D, Dale DC, Omine M, Perry S & Wolff SM (1973) Periodic hematopoiesis in human cyclic neutropenia. *Journal of Clinical Investigation* **52**: 3220–3230.

Hall JG, Levin J, Kuhn JP, Ottenheimer EJ, van Berkum KAP & McKusick VA (1969) Thrombocytopenia with absent radius (TAR). *Medicine* **48**: 411–439.

Heimpel H (1977) Congenital dyserythropoietic anaemia, Type I. In Lewis SM & Verwilghen RL (eds) *Dyserythropoiesis*. pp 55–70. London: Academic Press.

Heimpel H & Wendt F (1968) Congenital dyserythropoietic anaemia with karyorrhexis and multinuclearity of normoblasts. *Helvetica Medica Acta* **34**: 103–115.

Hinchcliffe RF & Lilleyman JS (1987) *Practial Paediatric Haematology*. Chichester: John Wiley and Sons Ltd.

Howe RB, Branda RF, Douglas SD & Brunning RD (1979) Hereditary dyserythropoiesis with abnormal membrane folate transport. *Blood* **54**: 1080–1090.

Kawaguchi Y, Kobayashi M, Tanabe A et al (1985) Granulopoiesis in patients with congenital neutropenia. *American Journal of Hematology* **20**: 223–234.

Kenney D, Cairns L, Remold-O'Donnell E, Peterson J, Rosen FS & Parkman R (1986) Morphological abnormalities in the lymphocytes of patients with the Wiskott–Aldrich syndrome. *Blood* **68**: 1329–1332.

Kenny MW, Ibbotson RM, Hand MJ & Tector MJ (1978) Congenital dyserythropoietic anaemia with unusual cytoplasmic inclusions. *Journal of Clinical Pathology* **31**: 1228–1233.

Kinugawa N & Ohtani T (1985) Beneficial effects of high-dose intravenous gammaglobulin on the accelerated phase of Chediak–Higashi syndrome. *Helvetica Paediatrica Acta* **40**: 169–172.

Kostmann R (1956) Infantile genetic agranulocytosis. *Acta Paediatrica* **45(supplement 105)**: 1–78.

Kostmann R (1975) Infantile genetic agranulocytosis. A review with presentation of ten new cases. *Acta Paediatrica Scandinavica* **64**: 362–368.

Lange RD & Jones JB (1987) Cyclic neutropenia: review of clinical manifestations and management. *American Journal of Pediatric Hematology/Oncology* **3**: 363–367.

Lenarsky C, Weinberg K, Guinan E et al (1988) Bone marrow transplantation for constitutional red cell aplasia. *Blood* **71**: 226–229.

Lightsey AL, Parmley RT, Marsh WL et al (1985) Severe congenital neutropenia with unique features of dysgranulopoiesis. *American Journal of Hematology* **18**: 59–71.

Lowenthal RM, Marsden KA, Dewar CL & Thompson GR (1980) Congenital dyserythropoietic anaemia (CDA) with severe gout, rare Kell phenotype and erythrocyte, granulocyte and platelet membrane reduplication: a new variant of CDA type II. *British Journal of Haematology* **44**: 211–220.

Marra G, Claris Appiani A, Romeo L et al (1986) Renal tubular acidosis in a case of Shwachman's syndrome. *Acta Paediatrica Scandinavica* **75**: 682–684.

Mentzer WC & Johnston RB (1977) An unusual form of chronic neutropenia in a father and daughter with hypogammaglobulinaemia. *British Journal of Haematology* **36**: 313–322.

Mentzer WC, Wang WC & Diamond LK (1975) An abnormality of riboflavin metabolism in congenital hypoplastic anaemia. *Blood* **46**: 1005.

Merino F, Amesty C, Henle W, Layrisse Z, Bianco N & Ramirez-Duque P (1986) Chediak–Higashi syndrome: immunological responses to Epstein–Barr virus studies in gene heterozygotes. *Journal of Clinical Immunology* **6**: 242–248.
Miller MR, Oski FA & Harris MB (1971) Lazy-leucocyte syndrome: a new disorder of neutrophil function. *Lancet* **i**: 665–669.
Miller AL, Stein R, Sundsmo M & Yeh RY (1986) Characterisation of lysosomes and lysosomal enzymes from Chediak–Higashi syndrome cultured fibroblasts. *Biochemical Journal* **238**: 589–595.
Morley AA, Carew JP & Baikie AG (1967) Familial cyclical neutropenia. *British Journal of Haematology* **13**: 719–738.
Myllyla G, Pelkonen R, Ikkala E & Jalahtiz APA (1967) Hereditary thrombocytopenia: report of three families. *Scandinavian Journal of Haematology* **4**: 441–452.
Nair MPN, Gray RH, Boxer LA & Schwartz SA (1987) Deficiency of inducible suppressor cell function in the Chediak–Higashi syndrome. *American Journal of Hematology* **26**: 55–66.
Nathan DG, Hillman DG, Chess L et al (1978) Normal erythropoietic helper T cells in congenital hypoplastic (Diamond–Blackfan) anaemia. *New England Journal of Medicine* **298**: 1049–1051.
O'Gorman-Hughes DW (1974) Aplastic anaemia in childhood III. Constitutional aplastic anaemia and related cytopenias. *Medical Journal of Australia* **1**: 51–52.
Ortega JA & Lazerson J (1987) Anagyrine-induced red cell aplasia, vascular anomaly, and skeletal dysplasia. *Journal of Pediatrics* **111**: 87–89.
Ozsoylu S (1984) Bolus methyl prednisolone for refractory Diamond–Blackfan syndrome. *Lancet* **ii**: 1033.
Parmley RT, Crist WM, Ragab AH et al (1980) Congenital dysgranulopoietic neutropenia: clinical, serologic and in vitro proliferative characteristics. *Blood* **56**: 465–475.
Peacocke M & Simanovitch KA (1987) Linkage of the Wiskott–Aldrich syndrome with polymorphic DNA sequences from the human X chromosome. *Proceedings of the National Academy of Sciences of the USA* **84**: 3430–3433.
Price TH & Dale DC (1978) The selective neutropenias. *Clinics in Haematology* **7**: 501–521.
Remold-O'Donnell E, Kenney DM, Parkman R, Cairns L, Savage B & Rosen FS (1984) Characterisation of a human lymphocyte surface sialoglycoprotein that is defective in Wiskott–Aldrich syndrome. *Journal of Experimental Medicine* **159**: 1705.
Remold-O'Donnell E, Zimmerman C, Kenney D & Rosen FS (1987) Expression on blood cells of sialophorin, the surface glycoprotein that is defective in Wiskott–Aldrich syndrome. *Blood* **70**: 104–109.
Rothbaum RJ, Williams DA & Daugherty CC (1982) Unusual surface distribution of concanavalin A reflects a cytoskeletal defect in Shwachman's syndrome. *Lancet* **ii**: 800–801.
Saunders EF & Freedman MH (1978) Constitutional aplastic anaemia: defective haemopoietic stem cell growth *in vitro*. *British Journal of Haematology* **40**: 277–287.
Shmerling DH, Prader A, Hitzig WH, Giedion A, Hadorn B & Kuhni M (1969) The syndrome of exocrine pancreatic insufficiency, neutropenia, metaphyseal dysostosis and dwarfism. *Helvetica Paediatrica Acta* **24**: 547–575.
Shwachman H, Diamond LK, Oski FA & Khan A-T (1964) The syndrome of pancreatic insufficiency and bone marrow dysfunction. *Journal of Pediatrics* **65**: 645–663.
Standen GR, Lillicrap DP, Matthews N & Bloom AL (1986) Inherited thrombocytopenia, elevated serum IgA and renal disease: identification as a variant of the Wiskott–Aldrich syndrome. *Quarterly Journal of Medicine* **59**: 401–408.
Standen GR (1988) Wiskott–Aldrich syndrome: new perspectives in pathogenesis and management. *Journal of the Royal College of Physicians of London* **22**: 80–83.
Steinberg MH, Coleman MF & Pennebaker JB (1979) Diamond–Blackfan syndrome: evidence for T-cell mediated suppression of erythroid development and a serum blocking factor associated with remission. *British Journal of Haematology* **41**: 57–68.
Stuart MJ & McKenna R (1981) Diseases of coagulation: the platelet and vasculature. In Nathan DG & Oski FA (eds) *Hematology of Infancy and Childhood*, 2nd edn., pp 1234–1338. Philadelphia: WB Saunders.
Szüts P, Katona Z, Ilyes M, Szabo I & Czato M (1984) Correction of defective chemotaxis with thiamine in Shwachman–Diamond syndrome. *Lancet* **i**: 1072–1073.

Tötterman TH, Nisell J, Killander A, Gahrton G & Lönnqvist B (1984) Successful treatment of pure red-cell aplasia with cyclosporin. *Lancet* **ii**: 693.

Verwilghen RL, Lewis SM, Dacie JV, Crookston JH & Crookston MC (1973) HEMPAS: Congenital dyserythropoietic anaemia (type II). *Quarterly Journal of Medicine:* **42**: 257–278.

von Schulthess GK, Fehr J & Dahinden C (1983) Cyclic neutropenia: amplification of granulocyte oscillations by lithium and long-term suppression of cycling by plasmapheresis. *Blood* **62**: 320–326.

Weiden PL, Robinette B, Adamson JW, Graham TC & Storb R (1973) Marrow transplantation in canine cyclic neutropenia. *Blood* **42**: 1009.

Whitefield MF & Barr DGD (1976) Cows milk allergy in the syndrome of thrombocytopenia with absent radius. *Archives of disease in Childhood* **51**: 337–343.

Whitehouse DB, Hopkinson DA & Evans DIK (1984) Adenosine deaminase activity in Diamond–Blackfan syndrome. *Lancet* **ii**: 1398–1399.

Wright DG, Fauci AS, Dale DC & Wolff SM (1978) Correction of human cyclic neutropenia with prednisolone. *New England Journal of Medicine* **298**: 295–300.

Zucker-Franklin D, L'Esperance P & Good RA (1977) Congenital neutropenia: an intrinsic cell defect demonstrated by electron microscopy of soft agar colonies. *Blood* **49**: 425–436.

Zuelzer WW (1964) Myelokathexis—a new form of chronic granulocytopenia. *New England Journal of Medicine* **270**: 699–704.

Index

Note: Page numbers of article titles are in **bold** type.